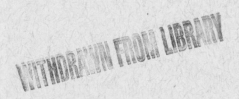

Making Miracles: In Vitro Fertilization

Books by Nan and Todd Tilton and Gaylen Moore:

MAKING MIRACLES: IN VITRO FERTILIZATION

Also by Gaylen Moore:

PARTICULAR PASSIONS: TALKS WITH WOMEN WHO
HAVE SHAPED OUR TIMES by Lynn Gilbert and Gaylen Moore

Making Miracles:
In Vitro Fertilization

Nan and Todd Tilton
and Gaylen Moore

Doubleday & Company, Inc., Garden City, New York   1985

Some of the names in *Making Miracles: In Vitro Fertilization* are fictitious, to protect the anonymity of those individuals.

"Minimal Standards for Programs of In Vitro Fertilization" is reprinted from *Fertility and Sterility*, Volume 41, No. 1, January 1984, copyright © 1984 by The American Fertility Society. Reproduced by permission of the publisher, The American Fertility Society, Birmingham, Alabama.

Library of Congress Cataloging in Publication Data
Tilton, Nan.
　Making miracles.
　Includes index.
　1. Fertilization in vitro, Human.　2. Tilton, Nan.
3. Pregnant women—United States—Biography.　4. Twins—
United States—Biography.　I. Tilton, Todd.　II. Moore,
Gaylen.　III. Title.
RG135.T55　1985　　618.1'78

We would like to express our gratitude to Dr. Howard Jones, Jr.; Dr. Georgeanna Seegar Jones; Dr. Jairo Garcia; and the entire in vitro team at the Howard and Georgeanna Jones Institute for Reproductive Medicine. To Dr. Paul Mazzarella, our obstetrician; Dr. Michael Gilbert, our pediatrician; and the many other doctors who helped us, thank you.

To those couples still waiting, we send our message of hope.

Preface

Infertility is not fatal—or is it? For some couples, childbearing is an expected and almost required event. Why? The reasons vary—perhaps for cultural and family reasons, perhaps for love of children, perhaps from guilt over a transgression thought to have caused the infertility problem, perhaps as the ultimate expression of devotion. But for whatever reason, or combinations of reasons, having a child is, for many couples, a requirement for the fulfillment of life. If this expectation is shattered and the ideal becomes unattainable, it can become necessary for the couple to redefine the meaning of life together.

For some couples this may be easy. Others, when faced with infertility, quickly focus on alternative goals. For still others, reproductive failure is devastating. Infertility often comes as a special shock to those who have postponed their family, not realizing that reproduction is sensitive to age and disease.

And so, is infertility fatal? Not in the literal sense, of course. Nevertheless, for some couples the shattering of childhood dreams and youthful expectations may leave a scar that disfigures life forever.

The story of Nan and Todd Tilton should give hope to infertile couples who have failed to benefit from any form of conventional therapy. In vitro fertilization is an exhausting and consuming experience for the couple (and, we might say, for the medical team). It requires motivation, determination, and endurance. Its failures are more frequent than its successes and they weigh heavily on us all. Nevertheless, improvement is occurring across the country and around the world. Furthermore, in vitro fertilization for the first time has provided the opportunity to observe facets of human reproduction never before examined. Thus, there is the opportunity to fill in and understand these blank areas. This new information, this spin-off from in vitro fertilization, is already being applied to other fields of reproduction.

Medical science can progress only so far in the laboratory. There comes a time when there is no substitute for a clinical trial. This requires daring people who are willing to be partners in a venture with an uncertain outcome. The story of Nan and Todd Tilton is therefore not only the story of in vitro fertilization, it is also the story of the brave partnership between patient and a carefully conceived clinical concept so necessary to make tomorrow better than today.

—Howard W. Jones, Jr., M.D.

—Georgeanna Seegar Jones, M.D.

Founders of the Howard and Georgeanna Jones Institute for Reproductive Medicine, Eastern Virginia Medical School, Norfolk, Virginia

Contents

PREFACE   ix
1. The Infertility Experience   1
2. Todd's Problem   15
3. Nan's Problem   29
4. In Vitro Fertilization   48
5. The Screening   67
6. In Vitro Fertilization Begins   83
7. Laparoscopy and Transfer   106
8. Pregnancy and Birth   126
9. One Year Later   147
   APPENDIX A In Vitro Fertilization Programs in the United States and the World   161
   APPENDIX B Minimal Standards for Programs of In Vitro Fertilization   189
   INDEX   191

Making Miracles: In Vitro Fertilization

1

The Infertility Experience

On Friday, July 2, 1982, Nancy Tilton got her period. She woke up with it.

Before she got out of bed, she did two things. She marked her period on a basal temperature chart as she had been doing off and on since 1978. "We could wallpaper a house with those charts," says her husband, Todd Tilton. Then Nancy called Linda Lynch, the administrative assistant of the Vital Initiation of Pregnancy Program at the Eastern Virginia Medical School in Norfolk, Virginia. "Linda," said Nan, "I got my period."

"Come on down," Linda said. "We're waiting for you. We'll see you Sunday morning at eight, Room 304 Medical Tower."

Nancy Tilton gave a dinner party that night for four friends. Chicken thighs marinated in soy sauce, spaghetti, salad, blueberry dessert—it all turned out perfectly. Nan took pleasure in her ability to plan and cook a good meal. "It's a means of artistic expression," she says, "to be able to create an atmosphere in which people enjoy each other."

Everyone had a good time that night. Nan laughed with her guests, Todd kept the drinks coming—for them, not for Nan or himself—and all the time, Nan was thinking about just one thing.

For the first time since she and Todd had discovered in 1978 that they had infertility problems, they had reason to hope they might be able to conceive their very own child. In two days, she and Todd were going to be offered the very best chance that medical science could give them to have a baby. Not a baby conceived by artificial insemination with Nan's egg and donor sperm, but a baby conceived with Nan's egg and Todd's sperm, in the procedure called in vitro fertilization. They would have what is more commonly known as a test-tube baby.

Nan's egg would be fertilized with Todd's sperm in a glass petri dish in the laboratory, and the developing embryo would be inserted directly into Nan's uterus. If they were lucky, Nan would carry the embryo to term and deliver a normal, healthy baby.

Nan and Todd knew there was no guarantee that in vitro fertilization would work for them. In July 1982, the chances of achieving pregnancy with the in vitro procedure, at the Eastern Virginia Medical School VIP Program, were very slim, only 18 percent. But Nan and Todd Tilton didn't care. The odds against their having a child had been so much worse.

An estimated 3.5 million couples in the United States are infertile—1 in every 8 couples. A couple is designated infertile if after a year of trying, pregnancy has not been achieved.

The causes of infertility are many. It has been established that female factors constitute 40 percent of the cases of infertility, male factors 40 percent, combined male and female factors 10 percent, and unexplained factors 10 percent.

According to The American Fertility Society, the two most common causes of female infertility are the failure of the ovary to release an egg (ovulation) due to irregularities in hormone production, and the formation of scar tissue on the ovaries or fallopian tubes, which prevents the egg from getting from the ovary into the fallopian tube where it can be fertilized.

A third, increasingly common cause of female infertility is endometriosis, a condition created by the overgrowth of uterine tissue outside the uterus in the abdominal cavity.

A less common condition of female infertility is an allergic or hostile reaction to the male partner's sperm. The cervical mucus kills the sperm once it has entered the vagina, preventing sperm from reaching the fallopian tubes.

The major cause of infertility in the male is faulty sperm. Either not enough sperm are produced by the testes to achieve fertilization, or the sperm that are produced have poor motility or are defective in structure, both of which make it impossible for the sperm to fertilize the egg. In some cases, low sperm production in the male may be caused by a condition called varicocele, varicose veins in the scrotum. Infections in the urinary tract can also reduce sperm production or sperm efficacy. A second and common cause of male infertility is an obstruction in the vas deferens, the duct that carries the sperm from the testes to the penis.

Surprisingly, the rate of infertility among couples in the United States has been rising steadily since the 1960s, and it has tripled in the last twenty years. The reasons for this infertility "epidemic" are unclear, although there are several factors which may contribute to the phenomenon.

One factor is the liberalization of sexual attitudes, which has led to more frequent sexual encounters and a greater number of sexual partners for both men and women. The consequence is a higher incidence of venereal infections, which have a particularly devastating effect on a woman's reproductive organs. Venereal infections can cause irreparable scarring of the fallopian tubes, ovaries, and uterus, preventing these organs from fulfilling their functions in the reproductive process. The recent widespread use of certain kinds of IUD contraceptive devices is also thought to contribute to the higher incidence of pelvic inflammatory disease which can cause infertility.

Another factor that contributes to the rising rate of infertility is that so many couples are postponing childbearing until their late thirties. A Yale University Medical School study has shown that after thirty-five years of age, the average time it takes a woman to conceive rises dramatically, from six months to two years.

Whatever the medical reasons for a couple's infertility, there is no doubt that the psychological effects of infertility are devastating. Infertility can influence a couple's relationship, an individual's self-esteem, and a person's ability to function effectively at work or at home. "You feel such a sense of loss," says Nan Tilton. "It's like being in a state of mourning. There isn't a day that goes by that you don't think about it. Some mornings I'd wake up and say, 'Today I won't think about it.' But I always did. I felt I wasn't normal. There was something broken in me, and it couldn't be fixed."

For four years, Nan and Todd Tilton had been living a life of growing despair. "It's not easy to believe you can never have your own children," says Nan. "You spend so many years trying not to have children. You don't accept the state of infertility the minute the doctor tells you. You keep thinking there will be a solution. The doctor will do something and then you'll get pregnant."

Nan and Todd Tilton's situation was complicated by the fact that their infertility problems were not accurately diagnosed until two and a half years after they consulted their first infertility specialist. For almost three years, they went from one doctor to another. Each doctor offered a solution, but the real problem went undiagnosed. Each new solution offered a fresh spurt of hope, but still Nan did not get pregnant. "Every

Thanksgiving and Christmas, we'd get together with Todd's family," says Nan, "and no kids again. Todd's two brothers were so prolific, they were already grandfathers."

It got so that just the sight of a pregnant woman made Nan cry. The Tiltons were embarrassed to tell anyone about their infertility, so it really hurt when Nan's women friends confided in her about their abortions, and the men teased Todd about wanting to prolong the honeymoon. "I felt more and more like a freak," says Nan. "I still wasn't resigned to the situation of infertility."

The symbol of Nan's hope was a photograph she had stuck in the corner of the mirror over her bureau. It was a photograph of Nan and Todd holding their godchild at her Christening. "Look at this," Nan would say, "it looks so right; it looks like our baby, doesn't it?" This photograph was Nan's talisman. It was the first thing she saw in the morning, the last thing she saw at night. "You become superstitious," says Nan. "I was convinced that thinking it hard enough would make it happen."

But with each new diagnosis and treatment, Nan and Todd's possibility of conceiving a child diminished. "You go rung by rung, down the infertility ladder of compromises," explains Nan. "You want a baby so badly that you find yourself considering all kinds of bizarre alternatives you thought you'd never ever accept. When we found out that Todd couldn't have children, I accepted the idea that I could have a baby by artificial insemination. Then when that didn't work, I thought, Well, how wonderful, I can adopt a white infant. When you find out that it's going to take seven years to adopt, you consider buying a baby, and you accept that too. You don't moan and groan because you can't have a baby this way or that way. It doesn't matter how you get it. You're saying, 'Thank God, I can get a *baby*.' "

Nancy and Todd Tilton had been married two years when Nan stopped using her diaphragm. In 1976, Nan was twenty-five; she was teaching art to elementary school children at Friends Academy, a private day school in Locust Valley, New York, not far from the Tiltons' home in Sea Cliff on Long Island. In the evenings Nan was taking courses toward her master's degree in photography at C. W. Post College. Todd was thirty-one; he had just gotten a new job as an accountant at Marine Midland Bank on Wall Street after three years with Arthur Young & Company, a Big Eight accounting firm. They had no reason at all to suspect they would have trouble having children. Both of them came from big families. Todd had three brothers, and Nancy had three brothers and a sister.

Nan and Todd had grown up on the North Shore of Long Island in the neighboring towns of Sea Cliff and Glenwood Landing. Todd's family ran the local butcher shop and market. Todd, like his two elder brothers, worked in the store summers and after school.

School was a hardship for Todd. He was in seventh grade when a teacher discovered he had a learning disability—dyslexia. "I'd been talking my way through school," says Todd. Mrs. Tilton got him a tutor and in six months he learned to read, but even today he relies on his abilities to listen, remember, and talk his way through to solutions, an ability which has stood him in good stead throughout the infertility experience.

Todd's verbal communication skills made him adept at serving the aristocratic clientele that spent the summers on the North Shore of Long Island, families like the Kennedys and Morgans. They ordered groceries by telephone. "I'd pick out the best crenshaw melons and lettuce for them," says Todd. "I'd deliver their orders to the house, and put the food away in the refrigerator." Todd's was the third generation in his family to serve the gentry. Both sets of grandparents, the Tiltons and the Macdonalds, had come from Ireland and Scotland to work on the estates of Long Island families.

Todd was the first in his family to go to college. "I went because I thought I could learn something that would help my father run his business," says Todd. Todd went to C. W. Post College and majored in accounting.

When Todd was a sophomore in 1965, he saw that many of his graduating fraternity brothers were being drafted and sent to Vietnam. Todd enlisted right away in the Marine Corps Platoon Leaders Class. Todd's family tried to dissuade him, but he was determined. "I wasn't going to be sent over to Vietnam as cannon fodder," says Todd. "I wanted to be well trained and go down fighting." He graduated in 1968 as a second lieutenant and was sent to Pensacola, Florida, for aviation training. He became a bombardier navigator, and a good one.

Todd was home on leave in November 1968 when he met Nancy Kellner. He went to his high school homecoming football game for old times' sake and saw Nancy standing on the sidelines, talking to the sister of a girl Todd had dated in college. Todd remembered seeing Nancy at the house when he'd gone to pick up the girl. Nancy had been fourteen years old then. "I always thought she would grow into something special," says Todd. "I wasn't disappointed." Nan's merry blue eyes and wide, full mouth, her streaked blond hair made her look like the quintessential American high school girl. She looks very much the same today. "And," says Todd, "she had a figure that wouldn't quit."

Nan remembered Todd too. Out of the corner of her eye, Nan saw Todd looking at her. "He was so beautiful," says Nan. "He looked so much older than the high school boys." Todd came over to talk to Nan. "We talked for a few minutes," says Nan, "gossiping about people we knew in common. Then Todd said good-bye. I don't know why I did it. It was just an impulse. I put my arms around him and kissed him hard on the mouth." Todd was taken completely by surprise. He told Nan he'd be seeing her at Christmas.

Todd flew back to Pensacola the next day. Nan got a letter from him the following week, commanding her to save every single day of her Christmas vacation for him. She did. They went out every night.

Nan wasn't what Todd had expected. He could never be sure what she was going to do or say. She made him laugh. "I tend to be predictable," says Todd. "Nan has an artistic temperament, I guess. It was good for me to be around someone like that. . . . I liked her," said Todd, "but I wasn't in love with her."

Nan fell in love with Todd immediately. "I'd been out with a lot of guys my own age," she says. "I fell in love easily, but within three weeks the guys eventually would turn into jerks. They wouldn't let me talk to another guy. Todd was older. He was interested in a lot of things. He cared about people. He was what I'd call a 'fine' person; that's the best word I could think of to describe him."

At age seventeen, Nancy Kellner was a girl who was surprising but who didn't want any surprises herself. She'd already had the biggest surprise she ever wanted. After twenty-nine years of marriage, her parents were in the process of getting a divorce. For Nan, there had been absolutely no warning.

Nan's father was a commodities trader and Brazilian coffee salesman. Nan and her brothers and sister had grown up in a house right on Long Island Sound. The Kellner children spent their summers swimming and sailing at the Sea Cliff Yacht Club. What Nan remembers most about her childhood were the parties—boating trips, dinner parties, picnics, people laughing and enjoying themselves. "We had so much fun, all of us together," says Nan. "My mother made it look so easy. I couldn't wait to grow up and have my own children."

That year their perfect family collapsed. For Nan it was a shock, a shock she still has not forgotten. It is an experience that has influenced almost everything she has done since then. There is a streak of wildness in her, of daredevil courage that she is afraid could lead her astray. She works to harness it, to channel it to her purposes, rather than let it work against her. In Todd, Nan saw the stability she needed to keep her on an even keel.

Nan graduated from high school in June 1969, and went to college the following September at the National College of Education in Evanston, Illinois. For as long as she could remember, as far back as nursery school, Nan had had a passion for drawing and painting. "I grew up through my drawing," says Nan. "I took risks there, I tried new things. It gave me the confidence to do these things in other areas of my life. I wanted to give other children that self-confidence."

Nan stayed in college only one semester. In April 1970, Todd got his orders to go overseas. Nan left Evanston and went down to the Marine Corps base at Cherry Point, North Carolina, where Todd was stationed, to spend the last few months with him. "I couldn't think about anything but Todd," says Nan. "I had to go. It was the time when three hundred and fifty Americans were getting shot or captured in Vietnam every week. Todd was going over there to die, I thought. I wanted to be with him."

Todd left for the Far East in June 1970. He was stationed in Iwakuni, Japan, waiting for orders to go into Vietnam, when he received word that his younger brother Keith had died. Todd was granted leave to come home from Japan for the funeral. While he was in New York, his squadron left for Vietnam. Todd finished out his stint overseas safe and sound on the ground in Japan and the Philippines.

"I've been blessed all along," says Todd. "I've always felt there's Somebody watching over me. I went through the war without ever having to kill anyone and I didn't have to die. I must have been doing something right." That's why, when his and Nan's infertility situation seemed most hopeless, he was willing to take the long odds and pursue the emotionally and financially costly in vitro process, because he was convinced that it was the solution for them.

Quite surprisingly, Nan did not rush into Todd's arms when he came home two years later in 1972. She had moved to Boston. She was renting an apartment with three girl friends and working at Peter Bent Brigham Hospital in the dialysis unit. In Boston, Nan felt free to give in to her wild streak. "I had a wonderful time," she says, her eyes shining at the memory. "I was going out with a lot of people. I wasn't ready to get married."

Todd was living at home in Glenwood Landing, working in his father's store; he was ready to get married. "Nan was having her fling up in Boston," says Todd. "She'd missed the chance to have one, going out with me. She needed to do it. I'd already had my fling. I felt it was time for me to settle down. If Nan wasn't ready to marry me, I was going to find someone who was."

It was Todd's mother who told Nan that Todd had a new girl friend. Todd's grandmother had died, and Nan had come home for the funeral. They had been very close. "I was in the kitchen at Todd's house," remembers Nan, "helping Todd's mother wash the dishes, and she said, 'If you want Todd, you'd better come home. He's seeing another girl seven nights a week.' "

Nan was surprised at how much the news bothered her. "I didn't think I wanted Todd anymore," says Nan, "but then when I thought of him married to someone else, I wanted him." Nan went back up to Boston. In two weeks she quit her job, packed up all her belongings, and came home to try to win Todd back.

Todd wasn't going to make it easy for her. "I liked the other girl very much," says Todd. "I didn't want to break her heart for nothing. I wanted Nan to be sure."

Nan was twenty-two years old. Back home in Sea Cliff, she realized she had spent the last two years of her life living for the moment. Somewhere along the way she had lost herself, her dreams, her ambitions. She didn't even know anymore what was important to her. One morning while she was brushing her teeth she heard someone on the "Today" show talking directly to her. "This is the only life you have," said the voice. "If you waste your time, you waste your life. You have to have goals . . ." Nan took her toothbrush with her into the living room to see who was talking. It was Alan Lakein, author of a new book called *How to Get Control of Your Time and Your Life*, published in 1973 by Peter H. Wyden, New York. "Things just don't happen to people," continued Lakein. "You have to work at them every day to make them happen." Nan finished getting dressed, went out to the car, drove to a bookstore, and bought the book.

That afternoon on the beach Nan wrote out a list of her goals. She still has the list she wrote on that summer day in 1973. At the top of the list, without even thinking, she wrote: "To be married to Todd." "That's the moment I realized I really wanted him," says Nan. "I wanted his children; I wanted his values. Todd and I were very different, but there was one fundamental thing we shared: a belief in God, a God you can turn to when you need help. I didn't know very many young people who believed that. Right then, that seemed like the most important thing in the world to me." Second on Nan's list was a job teaching art to children. Third was a house in Sea Cliff. And fourth was a family, "four beautiful, healthy, happy children."

That summer Nan went after the first two goals on her list with a vengeance. To get Todd, she showed him she had no intention of giving him up. She was there at his new apartment in Glen Cove in the morning when he got up, and she was there when he got home from work, when he got dressed to go out on his dates with the other girl. One night she was still there when he got home from his date. "She was sitting on my bed," said Todd. "She'd been asleep. I sat down beside her, she put her hand on my leg, and I knew—it was Nancy. Whatever she did, it worked." Todd and Nan were married a year and a half later.

As for Nan's number-two goal, a teaching job, she had continued her studies in early childhood education at C. W. Post College, "but teachers were a glut on the market then," says Nan. She took twenty-five extra credits so that she could graduate with a dual degree—elementary education and art education. She graduated in 1974 magna cum laude. Two weeks later Nan got a telephone call from one of her professors. "There's an opening for an elementary art teacher at Friends Academy," said the professor. For Nan, the telephone call was tangible evidence that her strategy for taking control of her life was working. "The professor could have called anyone in the class about the job, but she called me," said Nan. "I had helped to make that happen by being the best one in the class for that job."

Nan applied Lakein's principles next to preparing for the interview at Friends Academy. She got someone to help her write a professional resumé, then she had it offset-printed. She matted samples of her art work and made a portfolio. "I had all the answers," says Nan, "what kind of curriculum I'd set up, my teaching goals. Then I bought a new dress and had my nails and hair done."

Nan was hired almost on the spot. The principal at Friends Academy told her several years later, when she was promoted to director of the school's art program, that she had been one of the most conscientious job candidates he had ever interviewed. "I wanted that job," says Nan, "so I did what I had to do to get it." That was why, when doctor after doctor told her she would never be able to have her own children, Nan persisted when so many other women might have given up. "It wasn't going to work unless I made it work," says Nan.

Todd Tilton subscribed to the same philosophy. He arrived at this point of view at about the same time Nancy did. Todd was working in his father's market, making $10,000 a year. "I could have taken over Dad's business, but I didn't want to," says Todd. "I wanted an accounting job in New York City." Todd went back to C. W. Post College to take a night course in advanced accounting. It was being taught by one of his former professors. "He was a guy who had really helped me in college," says Todd. "He pulled it out of me, everything I had." Todd went to the professor one night after class and said, "I need a job. Can you help me get one?"

Todd's professor set up an interview for him the following week in New York City with Arthur Young & Company, one of the Big Eight accounting firms. "I knew about the Big Eight," says Todd, "the way you know about Harvard and Yale, but I didn't think I was Big Eight material." Todd went to the interview and was hired. "See?" says Todd. "Someone up there *was* watching out for me."

After three years at Arthur Young, auditing Fortune 500 firms and tabulating income taxes for some of their presidents, Todd adjusted to the fast pace of New York City. He wore the pink oxford cloth shirts and red suspenders his bosses wore, and he reflected their ambitions. His perspective on life had changed dramatically. "Now besides knowing what men like J. P. Morgan ate for dinner and what the insides of their houses looked like because I delivered their groceries," says Todd, "I knew how they did business. It made me realize that life is a business; it has to be managed."

Following the example of a former college roommate, Todd started investing in real estate. His first purchase was a two-family house in Glen Cove. He and Nan lived in one of the apartments in the house when they got married. Todd's second purchase was a four-family house in Port Washington. Todd's third investment was a seventy-year-old house in Sea Cliff. Nan and Todd moved into the house in Sea Cliff in 1979, and so the third goal on Nan's list had been achieved. At the same time she and Todd were working on Nan's fourth and final goal: "four beautiful, healthy, happy children."

That's when Nan began having this dream. "I'm looking at a beautiful black sailboat. It's early in the morning. First Todd comes up on deck. He's wearing a white fisherman's sweater because it's cool, it's September. He's out checking the lines. Then a little boy comes out. He's three years old or so, and a carbon copy of Todd, pale blond hair and baby blue eyes. He walks up and down the deck with his daddy. Then another little child comes out, and I come out behind. All four of us are wearing Irish fisher-man's sweaters. There we were, that was us, our family."

Nan and Todd had been married two years when they decided that it was time to have children. Nan had been using birth control pills for contraception in the beginning of their marriage, but they made her queasy and gave her headaches. She changed to a diaphragm, but after the pills it seemed awkward. She hadn't been conscientious about using it. "There were some months I was sure I was going to get pregnant," says Nan, "but I never did." Nan didn't think much about it then; she just thought she was lucky.

Nan and Todd Tilton stopped using birth control in November 1976. The first month went by, the second, the third. Nan did not get pregnant. Nan began to remember now the times she thought she should have gotten pregnant but didn't. She was a little worried but she put it out of her mind.

Theoretically, there was no reason for Nan to be concerned. The chance of pregnancy resulting from sexual intercourse during ovulation in normal fertile couples is, surprisingly, very low. There is only a less than 25 percent chance that pregnancy will occur in any one month's exposure. Therefore it is perfectly normal for a fertile couple to take up to a year to get pregnant. Within a year, 90 percent of normal fertile couples will achieve pregnancy.

In order for pregnancy to take place, four elements are required: There must be an egg, viable sperm, a way for the sperm and egg to meet, and a uterus to nourish the developing embryo. The process of fertiliza-tion is a delicate one, requiring careful timing. In the female, one egg is released approximately every twenty-eight days from one of her two ova-ries. A woman is born with all the eggs she will ever have. The egg that is released is one of four hundred eggs she will release during her lifetime.

At the start of the twenty-eight-day cycle, the pituitary gland, located in the brain, begins releasing a hormone called "follicle stimulating hor-mone" (FSH). Over a period of fourteen days the FSH stimulates one egg from among a huge pool to mature. As the egg matures, it forms a small blue bubble-like sac on the surface of the ovary. This sac is called a follicle, and the follicle produces two other hormones, estrogen, before the egg is released (ovulation), and progesterone, after ovulation. The function of these hormones is to prepare the cervix and the uterus for implantation. The release of estrogen from the follicle causes the opening of the cervix, at the end of the uterus, to become wider, and at the same time the thick mucus which covers the cervix thins out so that sperm can more easily gain access to the uterus.

Sometime after the twelfth to fourteenth day of the twenty-eight-day cycle, the estrogen being released by the follicle on the ovary triggers the release of another hormone from the pituitary gland, the "luteinizing hormone" (LH). The spurt of luteinizing hormone prompts the mature egg to burst from the surface of the ovary into the abdominal cavity. This is called "ovulation." Ovulation usually occurs between the fourteenth and seventeenth day of a twenty-eight-day cycle.

The egg is now in a sort of limbo inside the abdominal cavity. In order for the egg to meet the sperm, it must get into the fallopian tube. There are two fallopian tubes in the female body, one for each ovary. The end of each fallopian tube is called the fimbria. When ovulation occurs, the fimbria is wide open, ready to receive the egg. Millions of microscopic hairs called cilia located on the surface of the fimbria reach out and grab the egg as it is released from the ovary and draw it into the tube. Once it is inside, the cilia that line the fallopian tube move the egg through the tube toward the uterus. The egg is ready now to meet the sperm. The egg can be fertilized only within six to eight hours after it is released from the ovary.

In the male, as in the female, it is the pituitary gland which is responsible for releasing the hormones that govern the reproductive process. The pituitary gland in the male also secretes follicle stimulating hormone (FSH) and luteinizing hormone (LH). These hormones in the male stimulate a continual production of sperm in the testicles in 90-day cycles, at a temperature of 94 degrees. This is 4.6 degrees cooler than the normal body temperature. A higher temperature in the testicles will inhibit sperm production.

The sperm begin as germ cells inside microscopic tubes called seminiferous tubules. As the cells mature, they develop a head, called the acrosome, and a tail, which is what propels the sperm inside the vagina on their journey to the egg. In twelve days, the developing sperm move from the seminiferous tubules in the testicles through the small coiled tubes called the epididymis into the vas deferens, the male sperm duct. The vas deferens conducts the mature sperm to the seminal vesicles and prostate gland. The function of the vesicles and prostate is to contribute the fluid called semen that combines with the sperm when ejaculation occurs. If the mature sperm are not ejaculated within a month, they die.

During ejaculation in sexual intercourse, powerful muscular contractions push the semen into the urethra and out of the penis into the vagina. An average of over 100,000 million sperm may be released in one ejaculation. In order to fertilize an egg, the sperm must penetrate the barrier of cervical mucus covering the opening of the cervix and get into the uterus. They swim through the uterus and into the fallopian tube while the egg is there. Only one tenth of one percent of the sperm ejaculated into the vagina ever get into the uterus. Once they get inside the cervical canal, sperm are capable of fertilizing an egg for forty-eight hours.

No matter how many sperm succeed in getting into the fallopian tube, only one spermatozoa can fertilize an egg. To achieve fertilization the spermatozoa must penetrate several layers of protective membranes surrounding the egg. Once the spermatozoa has gotten inside, the egg and spermatozoa merge and no more sperm can get in. The fertilized egg now moves from the fallopian tube to the uterus, where it will implant in the lining of the uterus and the embryo will grow.

After the follicle on the ovary has released an egg, the ruptured follicle becomes a new endocrine gland called a "corpus luteum"; it manufactures the hormone progesterone. One purpose of progesterone is to close the opening of the cervix and thicken the cervical mucus, making the cervix once again impenetrable to sperm. Its other role is to soften the uterine lining, making it receptive to the implantation of the fertilized egg and preparing it to nourish the developing embryo should fertilization occur.

If the egg is not fertilized, the corpus luteum stops manufacturing progesterone ten to fourteen days after ovulation, and the soft lining is dispelled from the body along with the egg in the process called menstruation. If the egg is fertilized, the corpus luteum continues to produce progesterone for a while, in order to assure that the embryo remains in the uterus.

When Nan Tilton did not get pregnant after *four* months of trying, she went to the library to do some research on her own. She learned that by taking her temperature before she got out of bed every morning with a basal body thermometer, and recording it on a chart, both of which were available at pharmacies, Nan could pinpoint the day ovulation occurred in her monthly menstrual cycle, and enhance her chances of getting pregnant. A drop in temperature signals that ovulation has occurred. To achieve pregnancy, she and Todd would have to have sexual intercourse around those days so that Todd's sperm would be in the fallopian tube waiting when Nan's egg was released from the ovary.

For the next six months, Nan kept her temperature charts faithfully.

She discovered that she had a regular thirty-two-day menstrual cycle, and she was ovulating on the sixteenth day. She and Todd made sure they had sexual intercourse on the fourteenth and the fifteenth day of Nan's cycle, which was one and two days before Nan ovulated, based on her previous month's temperature chart. But at the end of the six months, Nan still had not become pregnant.

Nan remembers the exact moment she realized it was unusual to take so long to get pregnant. Her neighbor down the street had come over to Nan's apartment for coffee one morning. She was close to Nan's age; she and her husband did not have children yet either. She and Nan were sitting at the kitchen table talking, and in the course of their conversation, the woman mentioned she had had an abortion. "She was the third woman that week to tell me she'd had an abortion," says Nan. "All of a sudden it dawned on me. These women had had abortions because they'd gotten pregnant, because that was what was supposed to happen when you had sexual intercourse. You got pregnant. All these women were using birth control, and they had gotten pregnant anyway. That never happened to me. That's when I thought to myself, There's something wrong here."

That was the turning point for Nan. She stopped making rationalizations and started looking for answers. After two more months of trying, Nan made an appointment with Dr. Ernest Samuelson, an infertility specialist in Hempstead, Long Island. The earliest she could get an appointment was February.

2

Todd's Problem

Dr. Ernest Samuelson saw Nan and Todd Tilton in February 1978. Nan prepared for her appointment with Samuelson the way she had prepared for everything she had done in her life since she had read Alan Lakein's book—with the intention of achieving a specific goal. "I never doubted that there had to be something wrong with *me*," says Nan. "We were going to the doctor so that he could fix it." So Nan went to Samuelson armed with a detailed report of every symptom she'd ever had that might shed light on what she felt to be her and Todd's temporary difficulty in conceiving a child. But finding out what was wrong was going to require a lot more than Nan and Todd expected or were initially prepared to do.

Dr. Samuelson's designer-decorated offices gave the impression of a high-powered practice. It put off Todd right from the start. "I thought, This guy's seeing dollar signs for every couple who walks through the door," says Todd. In his appearance, Samuelson lived up to Todd's impression. He was expensively dressed, carefully manicured, and his approach smooth.

The first thing Samuelson did was to give Nan a pelvic exam. While he was examining her, Nan told him she sometimes had painful menstrual periods. She also recounted her history of "being lucky" and not getting pregnant when she thought she could have.

"That doesn't necessarily mean anything," Samuelson reassured her. "Your birth control method might have been working. What we're going to do is to work aggressively from now on to get you pregnant."

"I was so relieved," said Nan. "That was just what I wanted to hear." Samuelson told Nan to get dressed and come into his office.

Nan and Todd sat expectantly across the desk from Dr. Samuelson. "We were waiting for him to play God now," says Nan, "and give us the instant cure." But instead of a prescription to cure their infertility, Dr. Samuelson presented the Tiltons with a checklist of tests that had to be done on both of them, just to diagnose their infertility problem. "It was incredible," says Todd. "There were twelve tests on the list. It was going to take months to get through them." The last test on the list was a semen analysis. Todd said, "Stop right there. Let's do that one first, then we'll know if we have to do all those tests on Nan."

Dr. Samuelson put down the list and leaned back in his chair. "It isn't that simple," he said. "Infertility is a problem of the couple, not just one member of the couple. If we want to diagnose your infertility problem correctly, we must have as much information as possible about both of you." He recommended that Todd go for a semen analysis and Nan should have a laparoscopy.

Laparoscopy is the only comprehensive method of diagnosing most aspects of a woman's infertility. It is a surgical procedure done under general anesthesia, and it involves a small incision in the navel through which a miniature microscope is inserted. Through the microscope the doctor can observe the condition of a woman's ovaries, fallopian tubes, and uterus.

Dr. Samuelson was talking the Tiltons' language. Take control, manage your life, he was saying. Find out what the problem is, then solve it. But Nan and Todd didn't hear him. In reality, they weren't ready yet to acknowledge that they might have an infertility problem. "Surgery seemed too drastic to start off with," says Todd. "I suspected the guy was out to make an easy two grand."

"That was *too* aggressive for me," says Nan. "I wanted him to say, 'Go home, take your temperature for another two months and come back; we'll talk about it some more.'"

As Samuelson was talking to the Tiltons, his receptionist came into the office. "Excuse me, Doctor," she said. "What diagnosis should I put down for the Tiltons' hospital release forms?" Todd and Nan looked at each other. "Now I felt sure we were being railroaded," says Todd. "They were already drawing up the papers for Nan's surgery." Dr. Samuelson didn't even look up. "Endometriosis," he said brusquely. Nan's eyes widened in fear and she grabbed Todd's arm. On a snowy Christmas day the year before, Nan had seen her best friend, doubled over in pain from endometriosis, hobbling up their front walk on her husband's arm. She'd had drugs and surgery to treat it but nothing had worked.

Endometriosis is a common cause of female infertility; it is found in up to 20 percent of infertile women. It is a condition caused by the accumulation of uterine tissue outside the uterus, around the ovaries and fallopian tubes. Instead of being flushed from the body at the end of the monthly cycle, the endometrial lining of the uterus builds up in the abdominal cavity and grows there as though it were inside the uterus, causing considerable pain each month at the onset of menstruation. Treatment for endometriosis is not always successful. Some drugs are effective in arresting tissue growth in mild cases. Otherwise, surgery is required to remove the tissue, but there is no guarantee that either of these treatments will be successful in alleviating infertility. Only about 50 percent of the women treated for endometriosis become pregnant.

"When Nan heard Samuelson say 'endometriosis,'" remembers Todd, "she turned white. I thought she was going to faint." Dr. Samuelson appeared to be oblivious to Nan's reaction. He made an appointment for the Tiltons in a month to talk about Nan's surgery; and the visit was over.

By the time Nan and Todd got out to the parking lot, Nan was sobbing uncontrollably, and Todd was angry. "Where did this guy get off scaring Nan like that, with no explanations? I said to Nan, 'We're going back there to find out what the story is.'" The receptionist looked up in surprise when she saw the Tiltons reappear. "We want to talk to Dr. Samuelson right away," said Todd. "It's urgent."

Dr. Samuelson came to the door of his office and saw Nan in tears. "As you can see," said Todd, "my wife is very upset. You can't just throw out the word 'endometriosis' and not explain it. Does my wife have endometriosis or not?" "I won't know until I do the laparoscopy," said Dr. Samuelson impatiently. "Is there some reason to suspect she has it?" asked Todd. "I cannot say until I look inside her," said Dr. Samuelson. He explained that the hospital forms required a preliminary diagnosis before surgery could be scheduled. "We have to put down something to get you into the hospital."

Nan and Todd were not reassured. "I kept thinking, There must be something he isn't telling us," said Nan. This incident did not inspire the Tiltons' confidence in Dr. Samuelson. In some part of their minds, Nan and Todd had already decided, no matter what happened, they would not go back to him.

Todd Tilton scheduled his semen analysis with a urologist in Roslyn for the following Friday afternoon. He didn't go into the City that day. He spent the morning working at home. After lunch he drove over to the urologist's office. "We were going to tick off this test and go on to the next one," says Todd. At the doctor's office, the nurse gave Todd a little plastic container with a lid on it and a place for his name and the date. In the next few years, these plastic containers would become as commonplace to Todd as temperature charts would become to Nan. Todd collected a specimen and he gave it to the nurse.

The laboratory analyzed Todd's semen under a microscope. The technicians were looking at two things: the numerical concentration of sperm per milliliter of semen and the quality of the sperm. Was the sperm motile? Normal sperm move rapidly in a forward progressive direction. How did the sperm look? Normal sperm have oval heads and long tails. With the information the doctor gets from an analysis of a patient's semen, he can determine the man's role in a couple's infertility.

Todd read magazines in the waiting room until the nurse called him into the doctor's office. The doctor didn't waste time on the amenities. Todd heard the words he never in his life expected to hear. "Your sperm count is only slightly over 1 million, with very poor motility," said the doctor, "and you have pus in your sperm. I'm afraid you will never be able to have children."

Todd was too stunned to respond. It wasn't until after he'd left the urologist's office that he realized he had questions. "The guy didn't explain anything," says Todd. "He didn't say how many sperm you need to make your wife pregnant. All he said was that I could never have children. And on top of that, my sperm was infected. I had no idea what the pus in my sperm might be doing to Nan."

Todd's problem, low sperm count, is a common cause of male infertility. At one time it was thought that 60 million sperm per milliliter was the minimum number required to achieve pregnancy. But as the technology for analyzing sperm has become more sophisticated, more and more is being discovered about the role of sperm in the reproductive process. Today, doctors have learned that it is possible to achieve fertilization with as few as 20 million sperm per milliliter.

There are many explanations for a low sperm count. One of the most important requirements for the production of normal sperm is a congenial environment in the testicles, where the sperm is produced. The most important factor in this environment is the temperature. A temperature of 94 degrees, 4.6 degrees below the 98.6 normal body temperature, must be maintained in the testicles in order to produce sperm. A temperature higher than 94 degrees tends to inhibit the production of sperm. It is for this reason that the testicles are located outside the body, to keep them cool.

To maintain a temperature of 94 degrees, the scrotum has a regulating mechanism, like a thermostat, which compensates for too much heat or too much cold by pulling the testicles closer to the body in case of cold, and allowing the testicles to fall away from the body in case of too much heat. Some sources of heat can be eliminated; long or frequent hot baths, even the habit of wearing underwear which is too tight raises the temperature of the scrotum. Changing these conditions can sometimes restore the production of sperm to normal levels.

There are other things which are less easily eliminated, however, that raise the temperature in the scrotum. One of these is a condition called varicocele, which is varicose veins in the scrotum. According to Dr. Richard Amelar and Dr. Lawrence Dubin of the New York University School of Medicine, specialists in male infertility, varicocele is thought to be one of the most common causes of male infertility. Fifteen percent of men in the United States have this condition. It does not always lead to infertility, but it may, in some cases of male infertility, be a causal factor.

Varicose veins are caused by a malfunctioning of the valve in the veins which keeps the blood flowing through the body in one direction. When these valves don't work, blood can flow in the opposite direction, causing the vein to become enlarged. In the case of a varicose vein in the scrotum, Dr. Amelar and Dr. Dubin believe that warm blood coming from the kidneys flows backward into the testicle, raising the temperature of the scrotal sac and inhibiting sperm production.

Other factors which may contribute to a low sperm count are bacterial infections, such as mumps or venereal diseases, which can scar or atrophy the testicles. Poor nutrition, emotional stress, drugs, exposure to radiation—all these things too may have some effect on the production of sperm.

In Todd Tilton's case, the sperm count was so low that it was clear that the cause was more complex than emotional stress or too many hot baths. Todd's urologist referred him to a specialist in male infertility for further examination.

When Todd Tilton left the urologist's office that day, he thought, All the things people say about male infertility are true. "I felt awful," says Todd. But what concerned Todd more at that moment was Nan. Nan was standing over the sink at the kitchen window when Todd pulled into the driveway. He didn't get out of the car right away. Nan hadn't heard him drive up. She was always in her own world, making dinner; everything she did, she did with complete 100 percent concentration. She would never consider the possibility that Todd's visit to the urologist might not go well. It wasn't in her plan. She was the one who had the problem and the doctors were going to take care of it when they found out what it was. For the next few minutes, Nan's world was intact, her faith in Todd absolute. *He* was the solid one; he wouldn't let her down. Todd was about to put Nan's faith to the test, and he couldn't be sure, he realized, what the outcome would be.

Todd got out of the car and slammed the door. He knew there was nothing he could say. She would hate him, without wanting to, but she would.

Nan was washing lettuce when he came in. She looked up. "I'll never forget it," says Nan. "Todd's face was as white as a sheet."

"I can never have children," said Todd.

Nan stood frozen at the kitchen sink. "I was devastated," says Nan. "I felt as though I were watching this happen to someone else, not to me. All those months, not getting pregnant, it was Todd. It was Todd who couldn't have babies, not me. But it was Todd's babies I wanted."

Todd called Dr. Ernest Samuelson the next day to cancel their appointment. There was no reason for it now. Todd and Nan spent the weekend trying to be supportive of each other. Monday morning Todd went to work with relief. At least at the office, he was the same guy he was on Friday. He knew something about himself now he hadn't known then, but damned if anyone else was going to know it.

Nan went through the last three months of school in a daze. She woke up the first Monday morning of her summer vacation and didn't know what to do with herself. She hadn't signed up for any summer courses as she usually did because she'd planned to be pregnant that summer.

"Todd left very early in the mornings for work," remembers Nan, "and then all I had to do all day was prepare his dinner. I'd go to the supermarket to buy food and everywhere I looked there would be mothers and babies; I couldn't wait to get home. Finally I stopped going out at all. I spent the day worrying that I hadn't made the ice the right way for Todd's drinks and he'd be angry."

Nan didn't want to see any of her friends either. "If someone called on the telephone or came over to the house," says Nan, "I'd pretend I wasn't home. I'd crawl around the house so no one would see me through the windows." Just a month before, Nan had been driving to school every morning, singing. *"Singing,"* says Nan. "How many people love life so much that they go to work in the morning, singing? Now all I could think was, why bother to do anything, it's not going to work out. Nothing's ever going to get better."

Nan's transformation startled Todd. He came home in the evenings and found the house a mess and dinner not ready. "I'd never seen Nan like that," says Todd. "I kept thinking she'd get over it."

"Todd was shocked," says Nan. "He'd never seen anyone depressed before. In the Tilton family they don't get depressed. He told me to snap out of it. That was his way of dealing with my depression."

Weeks went by and Nan still did not snap out of it. Todd decided a change of scene would help. He planned a friendly weekend sailboat race on Long Island Sound with another couple. In reality, sailing was a solution for him, not Nan. For Todd, sailing was a microcosm of life. He set a goal, charted a course, and executed it with skill and imagination. He took satisfaction in rising to the challenge of the unexpected, taking risks and successfully guiding the boat to port. He felt masterful on his sailboat, in control of his life.

For Nan, sailing was something she'd always done. It meant good times and fun when she was a child, but as she grew up, she tired of the sailing life. "It's a very macho thing, sailing," Nan says. "There's a lot of beer drinking. The girls are all in bikinis; the men give orders." Sailing had been a way for Nan to be with Todd, to be his girl, to admire him. Going sailing was not the best solution at that time for Nan's state of mind. "I didn't want to take orders from Todd. I didn't want to have to bolster Todd's morale. I didn't care what he was going through; I was only thinking about myself. I felt so helpless, so powerless."

At the last minute, Todd invited his father to come along with them on the sailing trip. While this may have been Todd's way of escaping a confrontation with Nan, Nan did not consider Mr. Tilton's presence an intrusion. She was fond of him. Even now, when she is frustrated with Todd, or can't get through to him about something, she goes to Mr. Tilton to get him to talk to Todd.

The first day out, Nan fulfilled her duties on the sailboat without complaint, and the Tiltons beat the other couple to port. They tied up their boats at the Greenport Yacht Club, had hot showers, and changed for the big dinner that's as important a part of sailing as steering a good course. Nan was in agony the entire evening. She couldn't wait to get away from everyone and back to the boat.

The next morning, Todd and his father awakened early and went up on deck to wait for Nan so that they could all go to breakfast. They called down to Nan several times. Nan heard them, but no matter how hard she tried she could not get up. "I couldn't get my legs to move," said Nan. "I just wanted them to stop bothering me, and leave me alone."

Todd and Mr. Tilton went to breakfast without her. When they came back, Nan was in the same state. Todd was alarmed now at Nan's condition. Mr. Tilton thought Nan was upset because he had come with them on the trip. He didn't know, nor did Nan's parents or any of their friends know, about Todd's infertility. Nan and Todd didn't want to tell anyone. Todd's father thought it would be best if he went home. Todd took him to the train station, then went back to Nan.

Todd decided he had to get Nan off the sailboat. With a great deal of difficulty he managed to dress her and then he took her to a motel in the town of Greenport. Nan stayed there in the motel all by herself for two days with the shades pulled down. "I don't remember very much about it," says Nan, "except that everything was black." Todd called his friend Doug Hickock in Sea Cliff for help. Doug was the only person Todd knew who would understand what Nan was going through. It was his wife Sandra who had endometriosis. Doug and his wife had been seeing a psychotherapist about their infertility; Todd thought maybe their therapist could help Nan. Doug set up the appointment right away, then drove out to Greenport to pick up the Tiltons and take them home. Todd would go back later for the sailboat.

Deborah Goldstein, a psychiatric social worker, saw Nan alone once a week and saw Nan and Todd together once a week for the next three months. Deborah Goldstein worked with Nan to try to get her anger at Todd out into the open. Nan surprised herself. "I remember sitting in Deborah's office one day," says Nan, "screaming at Todd at the top of my lungs, 'I want a baby, I want a baby, goddamit, and you can't give me one.'"

Slowly, the worst of Nan's depression lifted. Still, Nan could not regain the confidence in Todd she'd once had. "I didn't trust him," says Nan. "I was suspicious of everything he did. He bought an apartment house and he didn't put my name on the papers. Suddenly I suspected him of ulterior motives. We had been banking his paycheck and living off mine. Now I thought it was because he had been planning to run off and leave me."

Deborah Goldstein's advice to Nan for the future was to take care not to get overtired. Everything she was going through would be exaggerated ten times if she weren't rested. "Deborah was a release valve for me," says Nan. "But I had to follow her orders." Deborah's orders for Todd were to stop drinking. As Nan improved, so did he. By September, Nan was ready to go back to her teaching job and she and Todd were ready to begin to try and find a solution to their infertility problem.

The Tiltons never went back to Dr. Ernest Samuelson. They were convinced that their infertility problem had been diagnosed. As a result, they missed the opportunity to get a comprehensive analysis of their infertility situation. This is a common error among infertile couples and one of the biggest obstacles to treating infertility successfully. If the Tiltons had gone back to Dr. Samuelson, they could have saved themselves three years of emotional anguish, financial expense, and a major surgical procedure. From then on, Nan and Todd Tilton took on the management of their infertility problem themselves.

On the advice of Todd's urologist, Nan and Todd Tilton made an appointment with Dr. Richard Amelar in New York City, one of the foremost authorities on male infertility. Before his first visit Todd was requested to report to Dr. Amelar's office on September 11 for a semen analysis. Nan and Todd were to abstain from sexual intercourse two to five days prior to providing the semen sample. "Even if a patient has had a semen analysis done elsewhere recently," explains Dr. Amelar, "we like to do at least one in our own laboratory when we start with a new patient. Each lab has its own way of measuring sperm." This semen analysis was to be the first of three analyses that Dr. Amelar required at monthly intervals. "Semen samples from the same patient may vary enormously from one month to the next," says Dr. Amelar. "We can't tell very much from only one analysis. We prefer to do three to get an average, and take into account variations with different periods of sexual abstinence."

The Tiltons' first appointment with Dr. Amelar was on September 26, 1978. Dr. Amelar is a genial, optimistic man. It was his business, he assured the Tiltons, to help get couples pregnant. A bulletin board in the waiting room, overflowing with birth announcements, was eloquent proof of his skill in enabling hundreds of childless couples to bear the children they thought they could never have.

Dr. Amelar first took Todd's medical history and then examined him. He checked Todd's weight, height, and blood pressure, and took a blood sample so that Todd's hormone levels could be measured. Then Dr. Amelar examined Todd for varicose veins in the scrotum. He asked Todd to close his nose and his mouth and bear down as if he were going to move his bowels. "This is known as the Valsalva maneuver," explains Dr. Amelar. "If the patient does have varicose spermatic veins, it becomes apparent in this straining movement. By putting my finger on the vein, I can detect an impulse of backward flow of blood going down the veins in the wrong direction."

Dr. Amelar found Todd Tilton to have varicose veins in both the left and right testicles. Amelar's colleague, Dr. Lawrence Dubin, confirmed the diagnosis—bilateral varicocele. "I didn't know if that was good or bad," says Todd. "If it could be fixed, it didn't seem all that bad." Todd got dressed then and went in to Dr. Amelar's office. Using diagrams, Dr. Amelar explained to Todd and Nan what a varicocele was and what role it is thought to play in reducing male fertility.

There is some evidence, say Dr. Amelar and Dr. Dubin in a paper published in *Symposium on Male Infertility for the Urologic Clinics of North America* (Volume 5, No. 3, October 1978), that varicocele is a condition created by the malfunctioning of the valves in the spermatic veins that causes the blood going through the veins to flow backward from the kidneys and adrenal glands into the testicles, raising the temperature of the scrotum, thereby inhibiting sperm production. It is believed that this blood carries a relatively high concentration of toxic metabolic substances, such as steroids, which can also inhibit sperm production.

The method used most frequently to treat varicocele is surgery. The surgical procedure used today is a modification of a previous method and was designed by Dr. Amelar and Dr. Dubin. The Amelar-Dubin procedure involves a small incision located a few inches above the scrotum, on both sides for a bilateral varicocele, on one side for a single varicocele. The vein is then tied off so that the blood flowing backward from the kidneys is prevented from entering the scrotum.

"When I get the results of Mr. Tilton's semen analysis and hormone tests," Dr. Amelar explained to the Tiltons, "I will be able to advise you on the value of varicocele surgery in your case." Nan and Todd made an appointment to return to Dr. Amelar in three weeks.

On October 17, 1978, Dr. Amelar presented the Tiltons with the results of Todd's tests. The first semen analysis showed Todd's sperm count to be 6 million per milliliter, slightly higher than the previous specimen taken by his urologist had indicated. "Less than 10 percent of Mr. Tilton's sperm were moving," noted Dr. Amelar, "and only 22 percent of the sperm were normally developed. There was no sign of any infection in Mr. Tilton's semen." The pus cells detected in the previous specimen were thought to be undeveloped sperm.

Two subsequent semen analyses showed Todd's sperm count to be no higher than 6 million per milliliter, with sperm moving not at all or moving sluggishly and with poor structural development. "In our experience," reports Dr. Amelar, "what is desirable to achieve pregnancy is a count of 40 million sperm per milliliter, with 60 percent of the sperm showing good movement with forward progression, and 60 percent with normal structural development. These numbers seem reasonable. Anything less than that, the chances of pregnancy are not as high. Below 10 million sperm per milliliter, the likelihood that pregnancy will occur is poor. But as long as a man has any sperm moving at all and they are well formed, pregnancy is theoretically possible."

Dr. Amelar found Todd's hormones to be on the low side of the normal range in both testosterone, the male hormone produced by the testicles, and the gonadotropins—follicle stimulating hormone (FSH) and luteinizing hormone (LH), the hormones released from the pituitary gland which govern the reproductive process. "I classified Todd Tilton as 'subfertile,' " says Dr. Amelar.

As a result of the semen analyses and the hormone tests, Dr. Amelar recommended that Todd undergo surgery to correct the varicocele condition, and that following the surgery he be given a course of injections of human chorionic gonadotropins.

"Before we decided to go through with the varicocele operation," says Todd, "we wanted to know what the surgery involved and what the chances were that it would make me fertile."

The varicocele surgery has been known to produce dramatic results in some cases. The operation has proved most successful for men with sperm counts, prior to surgery, of over 10 million per milliliter, according to a study done by Amelar and Dubin. The study showed that over a twelve-year period, from 1963 to 1975, in a sample of 986 men with varicoceles, 416 of them had sperm counts, prior to surgery, of over 10 million per milliliter. Of these men, 85 percent demonstrated an improvement in semen quality after surgery, and 70 percent of them were able to impregnate their partners.

For men like Todd Tilton with sperm counts of less than 10 million per milliliter, the results were less encouraging: 35 percent showed improved semen quality, and pregnancy resulted in only 27 percent of these cases. In an attempt to improve the semen quality of these men after varicocele surgery, Amelar treated them with injections of the hormone human chorionic gonadotropin (HCG). HCG in the male stimulates the testicles to produce testosterone, the male sex hormone. The hormone was administered by injection twice a week for ten weeks. Of those men treated with HCG, 55 percent showed improved sperm quality and 45 percent of these achieved pregnancy.

Those were the statistics that Dr. Amelar presented to Nan and Todd Tilton. "Based on these statistics," says Dr. Amelar, "the best advice I could give the Tiltons was that, while the odds were against their achieving pregnancy after the surgery, there was the possibility that there could be at least a partial improvement which might allow the use of insemination with the husband's sperm to increase the likelihood of pregnancy for them." The Tiltons did not hesitate. "That was enough of a chance for us," says Todd. "We would go for it."

The cost of the bilateral varicocele surgery in 1978 was a thousand dollars. Fortunately, with Nan and Todd both working, they had excellent insurance coverage. Todd's policy through Marine Midland Bank covered infertility treatment. "What my policy didn't cover," says Todd, "Nan's did."

Dr. Amelar performed the bilateral varicocele surgery on Todd Tilton the morning of November 15, 1978. It wasn't until Nan went to visit Todd in the hospital after the operation that she realized how far Todd was willing to go for them to be able to have their own baby. "He was so pale," says Nan, "I didn't recognize him. He had bandages all over his groin. They'd cut him up, his beautiful body. I couldn't believe I'd let him go through this. And I was so casual about it. I didn't even take a day off from work to go to the hospital with him. I let him go all alone, as he had wanted." That was the moment when Nan began to regain to some degree her trust in Todd.

Todd was required to stay in the hospital for two days after the operation. He was encouraged to get up as soon as he could and walk around his room. He would recover more quickly, Amelar told him. Todd couldn't wait to get out of the hospital. He walked conscientiously the first day; he went home the next morning with instructions not to exert himself for a week. As soon as Todd got home, he insisted on going sailing that very afternoon. "I felt great," says Todd. "The pain didn't bother me at all. I was already celebrating the success of the operation." Nan tried to dissuade him, but he wouldn't listen to her. She finally had to call Dr. Amelar to get him to talk to Todd. Amelar said it was common for patients to act this way after surgery. " 'Postoperative euphoria,' they call it," says Nan.

One week after the surgery, Dr. Amelar removed Todd's stitches and started him on a course of intramuscular HCG injections in the buttocks twice a week for ten weeks. "We look at semen specimens after the third month," says Amelar, "and then again at six months after the injections are completed. If there is any improvement in semen quality, it usually occurs within six months after treatment is completed."

Todd finished the series of hormone injections on February 1, 1979. Four months later, on June 8, 1979, Todd went to Dr. Amelar for a semen analysis. The results showed that there had been only scant improvement in his semen quality. "His sperm count was still very low," says Dr. Amelar, "but 20 percent of the sperm were moving now, and 40 percent were well developed. That was a 10 percent improvement in sperm motility, and almost a 29 percent improvement in sperm formation, after treatment." It still was not enough of an improvement to reverse Todd's sub-fertility.

"We gambled and lost," says Todd. And Nan and Todd listened as yet another doctor told them that they might never be able to have children of their own. Todd was beginning to consider the advantages of a life without children. "I looked at the couples we knew who had kids," he says. "They weren't having such a great time. Some of the kids were having problems in school or they were discipline problems. The children acted as a drag on the couple, holding them back." Todd thought of the things he and Nan could do without children. "I could get that thirty-foot sailboat," he said. "We would have time and the financial means to do some great things together. We'd have each other to think about."

Nan, though, was nowhere near accepting a life without children. Dr. Amelar suggested that she and Todd consider trying to conceive a child by "adopting a sperm."

"Adopting a sperm" is another term for artificial insemination. In artificial insemination, the sperm used to fertilize the woman's egg comes not from the husband, but from an anonymous donor. One day before the woman ovulates, the donor's sperm is inserted by syringe into the woman's vagina as close as possible to the opening of the cervix. From then on, nature takes over. The chance of pregnancy resulting with artificial insemination in any one month's exposure is the same as it would be had sexual intercourse taken place at the fertile time in a normally fertile couple, less than 25 percent. But of those couples deciding to have donor insemination 70 percent of the women get pregnant within six months.

"Take the burden off yourselves" said Dr. Amelar. "Start your family. Some couples do get pregnant on their own after they've conceived their first child by artificial insemination."

Todd's first reaction was "I don't want some other guy's sperm inside Nan." Dr. Amelar assured them that when Nan got pregnant, both of them would gradually think less about how the baby was conceived. "You'll go through the pregnancy and birth together," said Amelar. "By the time the baby is born, it will be your baby."

All Nan could think was, It's a *baby;* I can get a *baby.* Her voice trembles with the memory of her excitement. Nan rationalized the whole thing in an instant. "We would adopt a sperm just like we might adopt a baby," she said, "except that it was going to be at least half ours. Todd and I wouldn't be able to control all of the genetic part, but we could control the pregnancy. I'd have excellent gynecological care; I'd be eating the right things, and not smoking or drinking the way a pregnant teenager might who didn't know any better, and ate junk food for nine months, and gave her baby up for adoption . . ." Nan didn't see any reason *not* to do it. "Here we were now," says Nan, "on the next rung down from having our own baby, and I thought it was *great.*"

Todd admitted that the term "adopting a sperm" was a more acceptable way of thinking about the procedure than "artificial insemination." "It sounded much more human," says Todd. Some doctors who administer artificial insemination even mix the husband's sperm with the donor sperm so that there would always be an element of doubt; it might just be the husband's baby. But what finally convinced Todd to consent to artificial insemination was the fact that the procedure was performed without the knowledge of anyone but the couple and their doctor. Not even the doctor's receptionist knows. When the baby is born, it is legally the child of the husband and wife. On the birth certificate, the husband appears as the legal father of the child. "No one, not even our parents," said Todd, "would know it wasn't our baby. It would look like the varicocele operation had been a success."

After several months of weighing the pros and cons, the Tiltons made the decision to go ahead with the idea of adopting a sperm. Since the procedure required delicate timing, however, it was important that the Tiltons not have to drive an hour into New York City for their treatments. Nan made an appointment with Dr. Rachel Schachter, an obstetrician/gynecologist whose office was located in Rockville Centre, Long Island.

3

Nan's Problem

Nan Tilton made her first appointment with Dr. Rachel Schachter in September 1979. "I was very discreet about it on the telephone," says Nan. "I told the receptionist I was coming for an 'initial visit.' I didn't want *anyone*, not a living soul, to know we were doing artificial insemination."

Todd and Nan went to the first appointment together. For Nan, sitting in Dr. Schachter's waiting room was an excruciating experience. "It was full of pregnant women," says Nan, "and nothing to read but those sappy mothers' magazines with pages and pages of beaming mothers and cuddly babies."

Dr. Schachter was not at all what Nan expected. "She was very striking-looking," says Nan. "She had blond hair, which she wore in a French twist, and pearl earrings in her ears—very elegant." Dr. Schachter knew why the Tiltons had come to her, so she got straight to the point.

"One of my donors is a doctor who looks very much like Mr. Tilton," she said. "He's blond, blue-eyed, very attractive, and he has healthy children of his own . . ." Todd was thinking he hadn't expected things to be moving quite so fast. Nan was concentrating on the news that the donor had already produced healthy children of his own.

Dr. Schachter explained what the process of artificial insemination involved. Nan would have to begin taking her basal body temperature every morning again—rectally because it was more accurate—and record it on the chart for two consecutive menstrual cycles in order to be able to pinpoint exactly when she ovulated. On Nan's third menstrual cycle, Dr. Schachter would make the first artificial insemination attempt.

The sperm Dr. Schachter used for insemination, she told the Tiltons, was fresh sperm, less than thirty minutes old. It was collected by masturbation into a specimen jar. The donor must have abstained from sexual intercourse for at least two days prior to donating his semen. He was paid thirty dollars for his sperm, in cash. The majority of Dr. Schachter's do-

nors were residents and interns at the local hospital where she was affiliated as an obstetrician. They were men she knew through her work there.
Before she accepted any of them as donors, she took a medical history and
ran a test on their semen to ensure the efficacy of their sperm. As for
matching genetic characteristics, "I try to match eyes, hair, skin, blood
type as much as I can," said Dr. Schachter, "but it is often difficult on
short notice to get exactly what I want. I have to find a resident who is
free at the same time my patient is ready."

The cost of administering the artificial insemination in Dr.
Schachter's office was sixty dollars in 1979. This made the total cost of
each artificial insemination attempt ninety dollars, including the cost of
the sperm.

About the one thing that concerned the Tiltons most, Dr. Schachter
was adamant. "It is absolutely crucial," she said, "that you tell no one
about this, not your parents, not your best friend, no one. You don't want
someone saying something years from now that could hurt anyone. If no
one knows about it, then it can't slip out by accident." The only record of
the artificial insemination would be a consent form which Todd would
sign before the first attempt, stating that he was the legal guardian of the
child. "But this is confidential information," said Dr. Schachter. "On the
birth certificate, Mr. Tilton will be the legitimate father of the child."

The only question Nan had now about artificial insemination was
how long it would take to get pregnant. "You could get pregnant on the
first try," said Dr. Schachter, "or the third try. But it works. It takes about
nine months to a year to get pregnant with sexual intercourse in normal
couples; it's the same with artificial insemination if we do it every month.
Sometimes we might skip a month to see if the ovulation pattern is regular."

Todd still had doubts, but it was easy to rationalize them. He began
to think of this other guy's sperm as "medicine." "Nan was going to Dr.
Schachter to get the medicine she needed to get pregnant," says Todd.

Nan and Todd went home. That night Nan sat down on the floor of
the dining room with a year's worth of the big calendars she had thumb-
tacked in a row around the kitchen wall that she was using now to keep all
of her goals ever present before her eyes. "It's the only way I can see if I'm
getting where I want to go," says Nan. September, October, November,
December . . . "I mapped it all out," says Nan. "I was going to get
pregnant on such and such a day three months from then; that would be
December and I'd have a baby in September 1980."

That year Christmas with Todd's family was not quite as painful for

Nan. "Todd and I still didn't have a baby," says Nan, "but the next Christmas we would. I was sure of it." She was keeping her temperature charts with extreme rigor. The Tiltons decided that with all the pressure of the holidays, it would be better to wait until January to start the artificial insemination. "We thought we'd have a better chance of success," says Nan, "when we were relaxed and calm."

When Nan's fourth menstrual cycle began, Dr. Schachter told Nan to continue recording her temperature and to call her on the fifteenth day of her cycle to let her know what her temperature was. Nan's temperature usually ran at about 98 degrees until the sixteenth day when it dropped to 97.6 degrees.

On the morning of January 15, 1980, Nan was on her fifteenth day, one day before she was due to ovulate. Her temperature was still up, which meant that she hadn't ovulated. She called Dr. Schachter's office. "Dr. Schachter told me to say, 'The doctor asked me to call her today.' " The receptionist put Nan right through. The first thing Nan told Dr. Schachter when she came on the line was that she and Todd insisted they have a donor with blue eyes. "We won't take anything else," said Nan. Dr. Schachter told Nan to be in her office at noon for the artificial insemination.

Nan went to work and taught her first two classes. "I had to go to the principal to get permission to cancel my afternoon classes," says Nan. "He knew I was having infertility problems, so he didn't ask me any questions. I kept thinking, If he only knew where I was going. I was on my way to get pregnant."

Nan was going alone for the artificial insemination. There was no question of Todd's going with her. "I was very careful to keep a low profile with him about this," says Nan. "We didn't talk about it. I was going to the doctor for my medicine." As Nan drove over to Dr. Schachter's office, she was almost nonchalant. "There was none of that quiet desperation you feel when you come to the end of the line," says Nan. "I didn't know then that it was ever going to have to come to that."

Nan arrived at the office at noon on the dot. Dr. Schachter had told her not to wait in the waiting room, but to go in through a side door to an examining room and wait there. The nurse came in and told Nan to take off her clothes and lie down on the table. Nan had only been there a few minutes when Dr. Schachter came in with a syringe in her hand. "She didn't make a big deal about the syringe," says Nan. "She didn't hold it up and show me the semen or anything like that. You wouldn't have noticed it if you weren't thinking about it."

What Dr. Schachter did then was not unlike what takes place during a normal pelvic exam. With a speculum, she opened the vagina. She took a swab of Nan's cervical mucus and looked at it. She saw that Nan's mucus had all the characteristics that indicated the onset of ovulation. Just prior to ovulation, there is an increase in the quantity of cervical mucus. It changes from being translucent in color, becoming almost transparent. The texture of the cervical mucus also changes from its usual sticky and dense consistency and becomes almost pliable. The mucus at this time can be stretched out into a very thin thread without breaking. This characteristic of stretchability is called *spinnbarkheit*. All of these changes in the cervical mucus create an environment in the vagina which makes it easier for the sperm to get into the uterus.

After observing Nan's cervical mucus, Dr. Schachter was convinced that it was the right time to attempt artificial insemination. She took the syringe and inserted it into Nan's vagina, then expelled the donor sperm. "I usually put the sperm just at the opening of the cervix," explained Dr. Schachter, "or I put it just inside the lip of the cervix." She told Nan to lie still for twenty minutes to give the sperm time to get through the cervical mucus and into the uterus. While Nan was lying there, the doctor picked up Nan's temperature chart and drew a small line, marking the day of the cycle on which the artificial insemination was being administered. "I watched her," says Nan. "She didn't write 'artificial insemination' or put down anything on the chart that would give it away."

Half an hour later in her office, Dr. Schachter told Nan about the donor. "He has blue eyes and blond hair," she said, "and he's a really nice guy. He already has children of his own." Nan was pleased. "It was perfect," says Nan. Dr. Schachter told her to continue taking her temperature and recording it. If her temperature went up and stayed up after sixteen days, that probably meant she was pregnant. "That was all there was to it," says Nan. "It seemed so simple." Driving home in the car, Nan tried not to think about what had just happened. "It was too bizarre," she says.

The days passed; every little twinge or pain Nan interpreted as a sign of pregnancy. Her temperature continued to stay up. Nan's excitement began to grow, but she kept it to herself. "I was very subdued around Todd," Nan says. "I didn't want to rub it in. Todd and I were going to have the child that we both wanted and this was the way we were going to get it."

On the thirtieth day of her cycle, Nan got her period. "I hated the sight of that menstrual blood," says Nan. "It was another egg wasted, another baby not born." Nan had to wait until her eleven-thirty class was over to call Dr. Schachter. When the last second-grader had cleaned up his paper scraps, Nan ran to the telephone booth on the other side of the parking lot, by the maintenance shed. She'd found this phone booth when Todd was going through his infertility treatment. There was no one to overhear her, or even to see her there. She had absolute privacy. The booth kept her warm when it was cold, and there was a light for calls she made later in the day. She always kept a supply of change in her desk drawer.

Nan had only fifteen minutes before her next class started. She prayed Dr. Schachter would be there. She needed some reassurance. "Some women do get pregnant the first time," said Dr. Schachter when she came to the phone, "but it's rare." Nan felt better. She'd get pregnant the next time. She ran back to the art room just in time to greet the third-graders.

Nan told Todd when he came home from work that night that the artificial insemination hadn't worked. "So, try again," said Todd. Nan was glad he still wanted to go ahead with it. She could do it again with her mind at peace.

The next month, Nan was a little more realistic. "I thought that it might not work this time either, and we'd have to do it again. But I was angry. I wondered how many times I was going to have to go through this rigamarole before it would work." Every few days Nan called Dr. Schachter from her phone booth at school to report her temperature.

During one of these phone calls, the doctor mentioned she was having difficulty finding a donor with blue eyes this time. "My donors move on to other hospitals out of the area," said Dr. Schachter, "or they don't need the money anymore. Some will make exceptions. Sometimes a donor for a patient's first child will agree to be the donor for her second child several years later, even though he already has his own medical practice." Dr. Schachter asked Nan if she would take green eyes and brown hair this time.

Nan stood there out in the phone booth watching the time, wanting desperately to shout, "Are you crazy? Not in a million years." But she didn't. "What are you going to do?" says Nan. "You're looking at your temperature chart; you're about to ovulate. You want a baby. If I said 'no' and said 'no' too many times, maybe she wouldn't help us anymore. Or you're thinking, Not again, I have to pass up another month. It was taking so *long*. When you're living menstrual cycle to menstrual cycle, six months go by before you know it, then a year. I wanted to get on with it.

So I rationalized. I thought, Well, Todd's parents have brown hair and red hair; my hair is lightened blond, after all. But our kid has to have blue eyes. If it doesn't have blue eyes, it's not our kid."

Dr. Schachter found a donor with blue eyes. The fifteenth day of Nan's cycle came on a Saturday. Dr. Schachter told Nan to meet her at the office at three. This time Nan had to pick up the semen specimen herself. "We don't usually ask patients to pick up the semen specimen themselves the first time," says Dr. Schachter. "But once they're comfortable with the artificial insemination procedure, we do ask them to pick it up. It saves time and manpower."

The doctor instructed Nan to go to Long Island Jewish Hospital, to the reception desk, and ask for a package for Dr. Schachter. When Nan got there, the nurse handed her a Manila envelope with a lump in the middle. "She looked at me," says Nan, "and sort of grinned. She knew what was in that package." In the car, driving over to Schachter's office, Nan kept sneaking looks at the package lying beside her on the seat. "The contents of that envelope were just vibrating with life," says Nan. "Those sperm were swimming around in there, looking desperately for an egg. All I could think was, when they got inside me, they were going to make a baby."

As soon as Nan arrived at the office, Dr. Schachter checked Nan's temperature chart and her cervical mucus. The time was right. The doctor inserted the semen. Nan went home and she prayed. But the second artificial insemination attempt did not work either.

The third attempt was scheduled for March. Dr. Schachter was again having trouble finding a donor with blue eyes. By the time Nan reached the fourteenth day of her cycle, the doctor still hadn't found one. Nan, without consulting Todd, made the decision to skip March. She was counting now on April. In April, Dr. Schachter offered Nan blue eyes and red hair. "Todd's mother had red hair," said Nan. "I took it." After the third insemination, Nan left the doctor's office, hopeful once again.

Nan got her period two weeks later. She ran out to the phone booth to call Dr. Schachter after her second-graders had gone. "I'd made so many calls from that phone booth," says Nan, "and every time, the news was bad." While Nan waited, the nursery school children came out of their little brown-shingled house across the way to play in the playground. "They were so excited to be outside," says Nan. "They were just bursting with pent-up energy, running. It just wasn't fair. Why was it so hard for me and so easy for everyone else?" The tears ran down Nan's face.

"Nan?" said Dr. Schachter on the other end of the phone.

"It didn't work," said Nan, stammering, as she tried to hold back her tears.

"I can't believe it," said Dr. Schachter. "We hit it right on the nose every time. The mucus was right . . ." There was a silence. "I want you to make another appointment," said Dr. Schachter. "We're going to try blowing out your fallopian tubes, then we'll start the inseminations again. Lots of women get pregnant that way."

Nan went back to her art room to lay out the materials for the first-graders. She was doing collages with them that day, three-dimensional collages, with buttons, corks, beads, sequins. . . . She did everything in her power not to look out the window. It was the time of the day she hated most. The mothers were gathering in the parking lot to pick up their children at nursery school. Each mother went in and came out holding a child by the hand. "It was especially bad when it was raining," says Nan. "All the children wore those little yellow slickers and red boots. . . . I wanted to be one of the mothers so badly."

The next month, May 1980, Nan Tilton went to Dr. Schachter to have her tubes blown out. The purpose of the tubal insufflation test is to dislodge any temporary blockage in the fallopian tubes by blowing them out with carbon dioxide gas. It is a simple procedure which requires the patient to lie down on an examining table as in a normal pelvic exam. Under carefully monitored pressure, the gas is blown into the uterus by means of a narrow tube inserted through the cervix.

When Nan went into the examining room, she saw a boxlike machine with dials on it and next to it a tank of gas. Nan lay down on the examining table and Dr. Schachter inserted the cannula, then started the flow of carbon dioxide. "I didn't feel anything at first," says Nan. "I saw her sort of fiddling with the dials, as though the machine weren't working. And then it hurt, and it hurt and it hurt. . . . I was like a frog, my legs jumping, trying to climb away from her." Dr. Schachter turned off the gas and took out the cannula. "There's something wrong here," she said. "This procedure should not have been that painful. I'm afraid your fallopian tubes may be blocked."

Nan lay there on the table. "This was the first indication," says Nan, "that there was something wrong with *me*. But I didn't take it very seriously. I thought, Darn it, here's some new complication to hold things up." Dr. Schachter referred Nan to Dr. Philip Rice at the local hospital for a hysterosalpingogram, an X-ray of the uterus and fallopian tubes. "In some cases," said Dr. Schachter, "this test itself unblocks the tubes." Nan convinced herself that it would happen to her.

The only instruction Nan was given before she went for the test was that she was to bring someone with her to the hospital who could drive her home. "That should have tipped me off that this test wasn't going to be any piece of cake," says Nan, "but I wasn't prepared for it." The hysterosalpingogram turned out to be the most painful test Nan had to undergo in the entire four and a half years of her infertility treatment. "Women are always asking me," says Nan, "does in vitro fertilization hurt? I tell them that if they've survived the hysterosalpingogram, they can live through anything."

Nan's mother could not go with her because she worked, so Nan took her mother-in-law with her to the hospital. Mrs. Tilton was going to wait for Nan in the car in the parking lot. Nan reported to Radiology at the appointed time and was instructed to take off her clothes and put on a hospital gown. Then the nurse explained what was going to happen. "You're going to feel a pinch on your cervix," she said, "then you'll feel some pain, but you must lie very still." Nan wished then that she had had Todd come with her.

The nurse took Nan down the hall to a room that looked like an operating room. There was a large fluoroscope machine hanging from the ceiling, over a table. Nan lay down on her back on the table with her feet in stirrups. Dr. Rice came in and explained that he was going to inject some blue dye into her cervix. If there was nothing blocking her fallopian tubes, the dye should flow into the uterus and through the fallopian tubes, then spill out freely into the abdominal cavity. He would monitor the progress of the dye on a video screen by Nan's head.

Dr. Rice used a speculum to open Nan's vagina, then he inserted a long narrow tube about eighteen inches long, which held the dye. He tried once, then he tried again to get the tube into the opening of the cervix. "He kept poking and poking," said Nan. The doctor considered the possibility that there might be something defective in his instruments. He called for another cannula. It took so long for the nurse to get it, Dr. Rice was going to reschedule Nan's hysterosalpingogram. The nurse arrived then and the doctor tried it again. This time it worked. The doctor clamped the cervix closed. On a closed circuit television screen by Nan's head, the doctor watched the dye flow into Nan's uterus. He waited for a few minutes. Nan tried hard not to move. The doctor shook his head. "Nope, nope," he said, "the dye's not going through."

After twenty minutes, the dye still had not come out of the fallopian tubes. "I'm going to let you lie there for another twenty minutes," the doctor said, "to be sure." And then everyone left the room. Nan was frantic. "My mother-in-law was out in the car wondering what had happened to me. I was all alone. I prayed and prayed that the stuff would pass through the tubes." Twenty minutes later, Dr. Rice came back. There was no change. The blue dye was still stuck inside Nan's fallopian tubes. He said, "I'm sorry, Mrs. Tilton, both your fallopian tubes are blocked at the ends." The doctor then covered Nan with lead shields to protect the rest of her body and took an X-ray.

A nurse helped Nan get up and pointed the way to the room where Nan had left her clothes. Nan started slowly down the hall. "I could hardly walk," she remembers. "I got into the dressing room and saw all this blackish-brownish stuff coming out of me. There was no one to help me. I had to go out in the hall again to find someone who could give me a sanitary pad."

Somehow Nan got out to the car. Mrs. Tilton took her home to her house, put her to bed, brought her tea, and sat by her bedside the rest of the afternoon. "All I could do was cry," says Nan. "I was numb thinking about the consequences of the test and I felt so invaded."

The next day, Dr. Schachter confirmed the results of Nan's hysterosalpingogram: both fallopian tubes were blocked at the ends.

The hysterosalpingogram, however, is not a conclusive means of diagnosing blocked fallopian tubes. There are several factors which might prevent the dye from spilling into the abdominal cavity. There are valves between the uterus and fallopian tubes which act to slow down the sperm trying to reach the egg in the tube. These valves can close and prevent the dye from going into the fallopian tubes. If the patient is nervous, these valves might be affected, and the results might not prove accurate. For this reason, Dr. Schachter referred Nan to Dr. William Lipkin, a fertility specialist in Roslyn, Long Island, for a laparoscopy.

Laparoscopy. Nan remembered how she and Todd had refused to consider it two years before when Dr. Ernest Samuelson had recommended it. Had we wasted two years? thought Nan. "If I thought about it, it made me crazy."

It was only after the three artificial insemination attempts had failed, and Nan learned that her tubes might be blocked, that she confided in her mother about their decision to try artificial insemination. Her mother was shocked. "She didn't believe I could do such a thing," said Nan. Nan knew then she had been right not to tell her mother, or anyone about it.

A few days later, the consequences of the hysterosalpingogram hit Nan with full force. If her tubes *were* blocked, what were her chances of being able to get pregnant? Nan went to the library to find out. It was what she had suspected. Blocked fallopian tubes are a largely untreatable cause of female infertility. "For ovulation problems," says Nan, "they can give you drugs. For hormonal problems, sperm and vagina incompatibility, they can give you drugs. A tipped uterus, they do surgery; endometriosis, they can give you drugs or do surgery and maybe reverse the condition. If the husband's sperm doesn't work, you can have artificial insemination. But if you have blocked fallopian tubes, you're up a creek. There was nothing they could do."

She told Todd. He told her it was premature to foresee such dire consequences. "Don't worry until you have something real to worry about," said Todd. "We don't know anything until we see Dr. Lipkin." But that didn't stop Nan from thinking about it. A few weeks after the hysterosalpingogram, Nan made an appointment with Dr. Lipkin for June 4. That same week a Vietnamese family of seven came to live with Nan and Todd Tilton.

The idea had been both of theirs. "There was a time when every night on the evening news," says Todd, "there were stories about the Chinese and Vietnamese boat people. Nan and I kept talking about it, wondering if there were something we could do to help them." It was because Nan and Todd did not have children that they could even entertain the idea. Through Catholic Charities, the Tiltons filed a request to sponsor one of the displaced families. In May, the Tiltons received word that their application had been accepted. They would be sponsoring a family of seven, a mother and father, three children, the father's mother, and his mother's teenage daughter. The Tiltons arranged for the grandmother and the aunt to stay with a friend whose wife, Genevieve Sherwood, was Vietnamese. The other members of the family would stay with Nan and Todd. Genevieve would be their translator. By the end of the summer, Nan and Todd would have found jobs for the family and a place for them to live.

Nothing worked out as Nan and Todd planned. On May 16, the Tiltons went to Kennedy Airport to meet the Ling family. They were being flown in from Malaysia with a group of Vietnamese refugees. The Ling family was one of the last to get off the plane. They walked through the barrier looking dazed and confused. The children were quite young; there was a little girl six months old, and two boys, ages five and three. There was no question of separating the grandmother and aunt from the rest of the family. They wanted to stay together.

For the next seven months, the Ling family lived with Nan and Todd Tilton. Nan and Todd slept in one bedroom, and by choice, all seven

members of the Ling family slept together in another bedroom. Somehow
the Lings and Tiltons understood each other. Genevieve translated for
them at first, but after a while, they learned to communicate effectively
with gesture and facial expression. The housekeeping arrangements were
worked out by consensus. Nan did the food shopping and the Ling women
did the cooking. "It was much easier for Todd and me to adapt to their
food than it was for all seven of them to adapt to ours," said Nan.

No matter how difficult it was living with seven strangers from a
radically different culture, Nan was exhilarated those first few weeks. "We
had children in the house," says Nan. "Children. It made me feel almost
normal." She took them shopping for clothes; she found playmates for
them in the neighborhood. She enrolled the boys in day camp. Todd took
the boys sailing on weekends, and played ball with them in the backyard.
"Todd was great," says Nan. "They adored him; they called him Papa."
Before long the Tiltons decided it would be easier for the children to live
in this country if they had American names. So the children became
Brian, Jimmy, and Alexandria. As the summer wore on, and the Tiltons
became more attached to the children, they began to learn, painfully and
poignantly, what it was they were missing in their lives.

Neither Nan nor Todd were prepared for the way the Ling family
treated their children. "The cultural differences were extreme in this
case," says Nan. "Mr. Ling was always hitting the boys for no reason at all.
He slapped them on the ear, or the head, hard. We couldn't stand it."
Todd threatened to throw Mr. Ling out of the house if he didn't stop
doing it. He stopped.

Three weeks after the Vietnamese family arrived, Nan went to her
appointment with fertility specialist Dr. William Lipkin. While she was
waiting to see him, she got into a conversation with a woman in the
waiting room who told Nan that her older daughter had an infertility
problem, and her younger daughter had offered to have a baby for her. "It
was so weird," says Nan. "All these bizarre things people will do to have
babies start to seem normal when you think you're at the end of the line."

Dr. Lipkin called Nan into the examining room. He was a young man
with a ruddy complexion and an engaging grin. "He was very charming,"
Nan remembers. But she was not susceptible to his charms. She just
wanted a solution to her problem: how to have a baby. After Dr. Lipkin
had given her a pelvic exam, they went into his office. There on the
doctor's desk were photographs of his children. Nan found it offensive
that an infertility specialist could be so insensitive. How could he have any
idea of the pain I'm feeling? thought Nan. In silence, Dr. Lipkin looked

over Nan's file. He recommended that Nan have a laparoscopy so that the cause and extent of the blockage in her fallopian tubes could be determined.

Laparoscopy is a surgical procedure and it is performed under general anesthesia, but the patient is released from the hospital the same day. A small incision is made in the navel through which a miniature microscope is inserted. A laparoscopy can reveal problems in the reproductive organs which might cause infertility that cannot be detected by any other means, conditions such as scars or adhesions on the ovaries or fallopian tubes, or accumulations of uterine tissue which indicate endometriosis.

Nan brought up the question of endometriosis. "I couldn't stop thinking about what that guy Samuelson had said two years before," says Nan. Dr. Lipkin was noncommittal. "There's no way of knowing if you have endometriosis until we do the laparoscopy," he said. "There's no reason yet for you to be concerned. There are many things that can be done nowadays for blocked tubes." Nan wanted very much to believe him. She left Lipkin's office that day denying everything she had ever read about blocked tubes. "I had bad tubes," says Nan. "Lipkin was going to fix them." Dr. Lipkin scheduled Nan's laparoscopy for two months later.

June and July went by quickly. Todd went off to work early every morning, and the full burden of taking care of the Ling family fell upon Nan. Every day there was a new crisis, a new problem to be solved, new arguments to be invented to persuade the reluctant Lings to become self-sufficient. Nan was pushing, pushing herself twenty-four hours a day. Neither she nor Todd remembered Deborah Goldstein's warning—that as long as Nan didn't get overtired, she would be able to keep her depression at bay. Nan's mother remembered though. She came over one afternoon and found Nan in a state of extreme agitation. "I had huge circles under my eyes from not sleeping," says Nan. "I was thinking over and over, It's me, it's not Todd anymore, I'm the one who can't have children." The more she did for the Ling children, the more she felt that this was the role God had intended for her. Genevieve had told her that in the Asian culture, it is the role of barren women to care for the children of others. "Was this the closest I was going to come?" Nan asked herself. And she also asked God. The answer she kept getting was no. "I kept coming back to that photograph of Todd and me with the baby," says Nan. "We were meant to have children, I felt it."

At 5:30 A.M. on August 7, 1980, Todd drove Nan to North Shore University Hospital in Great Neck for her laparoscopy. "I'd packed a little suitcase," says Nan. "I could almost imagine that Todd and I were on the way to the hospital to have a baby. The only thing missing was the baby inside me." Three days before, Nan had had a preadmission work-up. They'd taken a blood sample, she'd signed admitting forms and filled out insurance forms then, so that she could go directly to surgery.

Nan changed into a hospital gown and got into a bed in Outpatient Surgery. There were seven other women in the room waiting to go to surgery. Several were undergoing sterilization; one had endometriosis. One by one the nurse gave them tranquilizers and wheeled them off on stretchers to the operating room. Nan was last. In the operating room, lying on the table, the last thing Nan saw was Dr. Lipkin, wearing a surgical mask, standing over her. He told her he'd be in the recovery room when she woke up to tell her what he'd found.

The next thing Nan knew, she was being lifted into a bed and Todd was there. "I tried to smile at him," says Nan, "and I threw up. The other girls were sitting up in their beds eating lunch; some of them were already getting dressed to go home, and I was so sick from the anesthesia, I could have died." Todd held her hand until she fell asleep again. Todd had left the room for a few minutes while Nan was dozing when Dr. Lipkin came over to her bed. "Mrs. Tilton," he said. "Mrs. Tilton, wake up, you do not have endometriosis. Your tubes are blocked and very badly scarred, but I can help you. What you have we can fix."

"Oh," said Nan, squeezing his hand. "You can fix it, you can fix it." She let the tears come. "Thank God," she whispered.

There was no good news though for the woman in the bed next to Nan's. Nan overheard Dr. Lipkin telling her that her endometriosis was so severe that it was threatening her life. She would have to have a hysterectomy. "That was the way it happened with infertility patients," Nan says. "You're like ducks sitting in a row, waiting to get shot down. You look around you and wonder who's going to be next, who's going to be the lucky one left standing. I was the lucky one that day."

Nan's condition, blocked fallopian tubes, is a common cause of female infertility. It affects an estimated 600,000 women in this country. In most cases, the blockage is caused by scarring as a result of infection. In 50 percent of the cases the original infection has gone undetected. In Nan's case, the cause of scarring was unknown. She remembers she had a fever and abdominal pain when she was a teenager. She thought it was appendicitis. Her doctor could find no cause for the pain, and within a week the fever and pain had subsided. It might have been this infection which consequently caused the scarring on Nan's fallopian tubes.

Blocked fallopian tubes is a severe form of infertility because it poses a serious impediment to fertilization. The role of the fallopian tubes is to grab the egg as it is released into the abdominal cavity from the ovary, and pull it inside where the sperm can fertilize it. This function is performed by millions of microscopic hairs called cilia, which are located on the surface of the fimbria at the end of the fallopian tubes, and line the inside of the tubes. These little hairs move at the rate of 1,200 times a minute to pull the egg into the tubes and transport it along to the uterus.

In order for the egg to meet the sperm in the fallopian tube, the tube must be open and unobstructed. If the tubes are scarred on the outside, the adhesions tend to imprison the fallopian tubes, and seriously hamper their ability to reach out and grab the egg as it is released from the ovary. This situation can be treated surgically. The scar tissue that has been holding down the tubes can be removed. When this condition is corrected, there is a 50 percent pregnancy rate.

If the scarring is located inside the fallopian tubes, however, there is a much smaller chance that the condition can be corrected surgically. In the majority of these cases, scarring is usually concentrated at the fimbria end of the tubes, near the ovaries, which may close off the fallopian tubes entirely. This blockage causes the tubes to swell up, and creates irreparable damage to the cilia in the lining of the tubes. This condition cannot so easily be treated by surgery. There is a surgical procedure which may temporarily reopen the ends of the fallopian tubes, but the chances of achieving pregnancy with this procedure are only 30 percent. If the scarring is located at the other end of the fallopian tubes, where the tubes connect to the uterus, the prospects for reversing infertility are much higher. With surgery, 80 percent of the cases result in pregnancy. From what Dr. Lipkin had said, Nan Tilton assumed that she had one of the less serious forms of scarring.

Nan Tilton left the hospital that afternoon. By that time her nausea and dizziness from the anesthesia had worn off. "I had to show them I could walk without falling down before they'd let me leave," says Nan. The next morning when Nan woke up at home in her own bed, the whole episode seemed like a dream. "I wasn't sure if Lipkin had really told me he could fix my blocked tubes, or I'd dreamed it." Nan knew she was being silly, but she wanted to call Dr. Lipkin and find out.

At five that afternoon, Dr. Lipkin returned her call. "What's the problem?" he asked. "Are you bleeding?" "I'm sorry to bother you," Nan said, "but I wanted to know. Did you say that what I had, you could fix?" "Yes, Mrs. Tilton," said Dr. Lipkin. "What you have is operable." He told

Nan to come back with Todd in a month to talk about it. "After we fix your tubes," he said, "I'll do the artificial insemination for you." Nan hung up the phone and whooped with joy.

The next few months were a busy time for Nan. On her wall calendar she recorded the important events. August 10, she was having a dinner party; August 28, Todd was taking Brian and Jimmy sailing; August 30, Nan and Todd were taking the children shopping for school clothes. On September 6, school started; September 10 was her appointment with Dr. Lipkin; October 22 Todd would take the sailboat out of the water for the winter. Then there was Thanksgiving and Christmas. She would have her corrective surgery done before Christmas, do the artificial insemination in the spring; in December 1981, she would have a baby.

Nan and Todd went together to Dr. Lipkin a month later. He examined Nan to make sure she had healed from the surgery, then he invited the Tiltons to come into a screening room next to his office. Nan and Todd were completely mystified. They watched as Dr. Lipkin fed a videocassette into a tape machine. On the television screen there appeared images of the female reproductive organs. "This is a videotape of a laparoscopy performed on a normal woman," explained Dr. Lipkin. He pointed out the ovaries, the fallopian tubes, the uterus. "Notice," he said, "how I can flip over the ovaries, get a good look at them all around. Now this is you," he said as another videotape came on the screen.

"It was horrible," says Nan. "There were these big stringy things all over everything. It almost made me sick to my stomach." "Those long stringy threads," said Dr. Lipkin, "are adhesions that are covering your ovaries. We can't even see your ovaries. The fallopian tube on the left side is blown up like a balloon and is lying on top of the left ovary, holding it down." Nan was absolutely shocked. She had expected to see only a little scarring at the ends of the tubes. This was a disaster.

Nan stood up. "You said you could fix it," she said in a steely voice. Todd put a restraining hand on her arm. "Take it easy, Nan," he said firmly, attempting to head off her outburst. Nan brushed his hand away. "There's no way you're going to be able to fix that mess," said Nan, gritting her teeth. Dr. Lipkin turned off the videotape. "Why don't we go back into my office," he said. He waited while Nan composed herself, then calmly, patiently he explained what he was going to do. The procedure would require two operations. In the first operation, he would insert two tiny plastic tubes in the end of both fallopian tubes which would open them up temporarily. Six months later, in a second operation, he would remove the plastic tubes; then the fallopian tubes would be open and ready to receive the egg when it was released from the ovary on her next menstrual cycle. When Nan had healed from this operation, he would attempt artificial insemination.

A glimmer of hope flashed through Nan's consciousness. Todd was immediately suspicious. "I'd already been that route," says Todd. "The gimmick surgery that got your hopes up, then the kiss off, 'Sorry, it didn't work for you.' I wasn't going to put Nan through that unless there was a pretty good chance the operations would work." He asked Dr. Lipkin, "What's the chance of success with this procedure?"

"I don't like to talk in terms of success rates," said Dr. Lipkin. "Sometimes I do this operation on a patient and I don't like the way it turns out, but the woman gets pregnant. Other times I think everything went perfectly, and the woman doesn't get pregnant. If you want my opinion, I think Mrs. Tilton's chances of getting pregnant after this surgery are about 10 percent."

Nan and Todd sat there, stunned. Todd was furious. "This guy had told us—not once, not twice, but three times—that he could fix what Nan had, and here he was proposing two major operations with only a 10 percent chance of getting pregnant . . ." "And that was still with artificial insemination," says Nan. "How could we, how could anyone put themselves through two major surgeries for such a small chance? It was insane. Besides, I didn't see how it could work. From what I'd read, I knew that opening the fallopian tubes wasn't going to be enough. There had to be all those little hairs to pull the egg in. Otherwise the egg would just float around inside the abdominal cavity."

This was the point at which Nan and Todd Tilton said, "No, this is as far as we'll go to give birth to a child. We will go no further." The Tiltons were lucky. Many infertile couples never reach that point. "I saw so many infertile women, later on," says Nan. "They went from doctor to doctor, trying anything and everything the doctors offered them. It was as if they'd lost their brains along with their fallopian tubes or something. They never stopped to think about what they were doing, or ask any questions. Todd and I were different."

"Remember," adds Todd, "we were managing our infertility problem ourselves. So we weren't afraid to ask questions. We were not going to let the doctors push us around. It surprised some of our doctors, I think."

Before Nan could bring herself to abandon her last bit of hope, she had one final question for Dr. Lipkin. "What about a test-tube baby?" she asked. "Would in vitro fertilization be a solution for us?"

What Nan knew about in vitro fertilization she had read in a book called *How to Get Pregnant* by Sherman J. Silber, M.D., published by Charles Scribner's Sons in 1980. The term "in vitro" means literally "in glass." The procedure called in vitro fertilization is the technique of bringing together an egg and sperm for fertilization in a glass petri dish in the laboratory. The in vitro technique then was only a few years old. It was developed in England by an obstetrician, Dr. Patrick Steptoe, and a physiologist, Dr. Robert Edwards, who achieved the first in vitro birth in July 1978.

The advantages of the in vitro procedure for infertile couples is that it does not require the egg to pass through the fallopian tubes to be fertilized. Eggs are retrieved directly from the woman's ovaries as they mature, and fertilized with the man's sperm in the laboratory. The embryos that may result are allowed to develop in the laboratory for up to forty-eight hours. They are then inserted directly into the woman's uterus, bypassing the fallopian tubes completely.

Silber pointed out in his book that the in vitro technique was particularly suitable for women like Nan Tilton whose infertility is caused by a blockage in the fallopian tubes that cannot be surgically corrected. But it is also a possible solution, Silber suggested, for men with low sperm counts. Bringing the sperm directly to the egg in a petri dish eliminates all of the obstacles in the vagina and uterus that sperm must overcome to reach the egg. Therefore a smaller number of sperm are required to fertilize an egg "in vitro" than would be necessary to fertilize an egg "in vivo."

Both of these factors suggested to Nan that in vitro fertilization might be a solution for her and Todd. Nan knew Steptoe and Edwards were doing the procedure in England. What Nan Tilton did not know was that the in vitro procedure at that time was still in the initial stages of experimentation. By September 1980, when the Tiltons consulted Dr. Lipkin about it, there had been only three in vitro births in the world. The chances of in vitro fertilization working for the Tiltons at that time were almost zero.

Nan and Todd Tilton sat across the desk from Dr. Lipkin and waited expectantly for his answer. "No," said Dr. Lipkin, "you are not candidates for the in vitro procedure." And that was the end of Nan and Todd's dream of ever having their own baby. "This was it," says Nan, "the end of the line for us. It was my problem standing in our way, not Todd's." Todd guided Nan out to the car. She couldn't see for the tears pouring out of her eyes.

The Tiltons left Dr. Lipkin's office that day with two different plans for the future. Todd was convinced it was time now for him and Nan to go on with their lives together. He had married Nan to be his partner, his business partner, his sailing partner, his dinner partner, his partner in the business of life, whatever it turned out to be. Their not being able to have children wasn't going to change that.

Nan, though, was not willing to give up her dream of the black sailboat. The little boy on deck would not be a carbon copy of Todd, but there could still be a little boy . . . if they adopted.

School started that week. Nan had enrolled Brian and Jimmy in the local public school, and found a nursery school for Alexandria. Nan was so grateful to go back to her teaching. Those few hours she spent with the children, even though they were other people's children, made her feel alive. "I saw the children thriving, growing in confidence every day because of my help. It literally kept me sane. Teaching gave me a way to express myself." Nan followed her lesson plan day by day by day and got through the fall.

In January 1981, Nan signed up for a course on adoption at C. W. Post College. "Here we were now," says Nan, "down yet another rung of the infertility ladder, and I was just as excited about the prospect of raising someone else's child as I'd been about having another man's child." Todd, though, had reservations about adoption. "I'd been reading those stories in the newspapers about the adopted people who were trying to track down their biological parents, and vice versa. It made me purple just thinking about it. If some guy turned up on my doorstep asking for his son after I'd raised him for eighteen years, I don't know what I would do. And if the boy I'd raised for eighteen years told me, he was sorry, he didn't want to hurt me, but he had to go look for his roots, I couldn't take it."

In spite of Todd's reservations, Nan threw herself into the adoption process as energetically and as thoroughly as she had pursued every medical procedure that might have improved her and Todd's fertility situation. But by the end of February, Nan had come to a dead end. It would take seven years at the very least to adopt a white infant through an agency. The only way to get around that was to buy a baby through a lawyer. "They call it the gray market," says Todd, "but it's a black market baby." The going price at that time for a white infant was $25,000. "It wasn't the money," said Todd. "I just could not stomach the idea of buying a human being."

When Todd objected so strongly, Nan did not pursue adoption any further. There remained one final alternative. Nan had been thinking about it for a while, but she'd been saving it for the time when she and Todd might indeed exhaust every other possibility. She broached the idea to Todd one night when they were in bed. "What would you say to adopting Brian, Jimmy, and Alexandria?" she said quietly. Todd was reading the newspaper; she thought he hadn't heard her and was about to repeat it when he answered, "I thought of the same thing myself." "We could give them so many opportunities the Lings couldn't give them," said Nan. "We'd pay for their education, give them a nice home . . ." Because Nan and Todd did not have children, they had no sense of what they were asking of the Ling family.

It was Todd who went to Mr. Ling with the proposal. "We thought he'd jump at the chance," said Todd. He did, but not the way the Tiltons had expected. He agreed right away to give them Alexandria, but the boys he would give them on loan until they were eighteen, then Mr. Ling wanted them back. "Of course he wanted them," said Todd bitterly. "They were his meal ticket." Nan and Todd did not even consider it. They wanted all three children or none at all. That was the end of the discussion.

Instead of transporting Nan to the brink of despair as she had anticipated, the realization that adoption too had failed provoked in Nan a feeling of immeasurable relief. "For the seven years of Todd's and my marriage," says Nan, "I'd been thinking, This isn't my real life; this is the interim before my real life starts. When I have a baby, *then* I'll be happy. I was finally coming to grips with the fact that I wouldn't have children. It was almost as though someone in the family had died. I went through a period of grieving. Gradually I came to accept my infertility and I had to go on and live my life. I had to learn to stop living in the future, and live in the present."

Nan was reaching the point of resolution. It does come eventually to the lucky ones. "For the first time in a long time," says Nan, "I could think clearly. I was optimistic about life. I began to see opportunities in my career . . ."

One night about a month later, Nan sat down on the dining room floor with her wall calendars and revised her life goals. By the same time next year, the restoration work on their house would be completed, she would have a master's degree in photography, and she and Todd would own a thirty-foot sailboat.

4

In Vitro Fertilization

One night Nan was cooking dinner in the kitchen, and she'd turned on the television in the living room as she always did so that she could hear the evening news. She was making white sauce. Todd didn't like lumpy white sauce, neither did she. Her attention was concentrated on the consistency of the flour and butter she was stirring in the pan when she heard the words "in vitro fertilization." She dropped the spoon and ran into the living room. From the commentator's closing comments, Nan gathered that a Right to Life group had been staging protests at a clinic in Virginia that was treating infertile couples with a procedure called in vitro fertilization.

In an instant, Nan forgot every effort she had made in the past months to accept her life without children. "It was like a bell to a Pavlovian dog," said Nan. "I realized that deep down I never really believed what Lipkin had told us. From everything I'd read, it seemed to me that in vitro fertilization could be a solution for us. I knew then that I couldn't give up the dream until I'd explored every last possibility." Nan didn't have a shred of information to go on, not a doctor's name, not the name of the clinic, not even the city in Virginia where the clinic was located, but she was going to find it.

The next day after school Nan drove over to the Glen Cove Library. By looking through the Guide to Periodical Literature and the New York *Times* Index, Nan found that the sole source of information about in vitro fertilization in the United States was one New York *Times* article that announced the appointment of Dr. Howard Jones, Jr., as the director of the Eastern Virginia Medical School's Vital Initiation of Pregnancy Program in Norfolk, Virginia, the first in vitro clinic to be established in the United States.

Nan gathered up her purse and a pencil and paper and went directly to the pay phone in the lobby of the library. She called Information in Norfolk, Virginia, and got the address and telephone number she was looking for: Dr. Howard Jones, Jr., 603 Medical Tower, Norfolk, Virginia. Nan chanted the address quietly to herself like a prayer, a mantra, over and over again. There was something magical and powerful about the words, Nan felt it instinctively.

She went back to the table and reread the New York *Times* article hungrily, desperate for more information. "There wasn't a single word about the in vitro procedure, what it was, who they were taking as patients," says Nan. She looked out the broad picture window of the library. The light of the cold February day was just beginning to fade. The lights had not yet been turned on. Outside, the snow was gray and the sky slate. Inside the carpet was gray too and muffled sound. Nan was alone. In the twilight of a despair she thought she had laid to rest, Nan wrote a letter to Dr. Jones.

Nan waited until Todd got home that night to tell him what she wanted to do. Would he go along with her one more time? "It made sense to me," says Todd. "I'd just read an article in *Business Week* on animal husbandry. In vitro fertilization worked with prize milk cows. From what I'd learned in high school biology, it seemed to me it ought to work just as well with humans. I also knew Nan would bother me about it for the next year if I didn't go along with it, so I said, 'Let's do it.' " That night Nan copied the letter she had drafted to Dr. Jones onto a piece of her stationery and on the way to school the next morning she mailed it.

That afternoon, as twelve o'clock approached, Nan didn't need a watch to tell her it was time for the mothers to pick up their children at the nursery school. She had the courage that day to look out the window, and she felt the stirrings of hope inside her once again. It was like rediscovering an old friend.

Nan figured that the earliest she could get a response from Norfolk would be a week, but it more likely would be two weeks before she heard from them. She wrote it down on her calendar: "Letter from Norfolk will come this week."

But it didn't come that week, nor the week after that. The anticipation was unbearable. One morning Nan could not bear the suspense a moment longer. She counted the minutes until the second-graders had finished their potato block prints. Nan had ten minutes. She put on her parka and dashed out to the phone booth by the maintenance shed, "her" phone booth, as she liked to call it.

"Dr. Jones's office," said a soft Southern voice at the other end of the line. "Linda Lynch speaking." "Hi, this is Nancy Tilton. Did you get my letter?" asked Nan. "I'm sorry," said Linda Lynch. "We receive so many applications; we can't answer all the letters right away. Before we can consider you as a candidate for our program, we must have a referral from your doctor. Ask your doctor to write to us, and I will bring your application to Dr. Jones's attention."

As soon as administrative assistant Linda Lynch hung up the telephone in Norfolk, she went straight to the VIP Program's files, found Nan Tilton's letter, and moved it to the file of current applications. "It was because she called us and was so nice on the telephone that I did that," says Linda Lynch.

Nan hung up the phone, giddy with relief. "They hadn't rejected us," says Nan, "at least not yet." She ran back to the art room for her twelve-thirty class, and for the rest of the afternoon, one part of her mind was on guiding the third-graders in the art of paper cutting, another part was on planning the strategy for her approach to the in vitro program. She definitely would not ask Dr. William Lipkin to refer them. She would ask Rachel Schachter. Nan was due for a Pap smear and checkup the following month anyway. She'd talk to Dr. Schachter about it then.

On March 6, 1981, Nan went to Dr. Schachter for a routine gynecological visit. After the examination, Nan got dressed and followed Dr. Schachter into her office. Nan had decided that she would not ask her if she thought in vitro could work for her and Todd. She'd just tell Dr. Schachter that they wanted to do it. "Todd and I want to go to the in vitro clinic in Norfolk," blurted Nan. "Will you refer us?"

Dr. Schachter leaned back in her leather chair, fingering the pearl earring in her left ear. Nan's stomach churned. Dr. Schachter studied her silently. "I know Dr. Jones," she said finally. "I studied with him at Johns Hopkins." Why hadn't she told the Tiltons about him, Nan wondered. "It's a very new thing, in vitro fertilization," said Dr. Schachter, "and very expensive. Can you afford it?" Nan had never thought about money. If they didn't have enough, they'd get it. "Will you write to them?" Nan insisted. Dr. Schachter picked up her pen right then and there and drafted the letter to Dr. Jones. What Dr. Schachter knew, but Nan Tilton did not know, was that the Eastern Virginia Medical School's in vitro program was beginning its second year of treating patients and had yet to achieve its first pregnancy.

The possibility of Nan and Todd being treated by in vitro fertilization did not even exist when they first suspected they had an infertility problem in 1978. It was in July of that same year that English gynecologist Patrick Steptoe and physiologist Robert Edwards presided over the birth of Louise Brown, the first human being conceived by in vitro fertilization. Her birth was the fruit of ten years of research in collaboration, and many more years of research before that on their own. These two men found in each other a common goal—to help infertile women conceive their own children. It was Robert Edwards, the physiologist, who gave a shape to their vision: fertilize an egg outside of the body and implant the embryo in the woman's uterus. It was Patrick Steptoe, the gynecologist, who provided the technique to realize their vision.

In Steptoe and Edwards' account of their discovery, *A Matter of Life,* * published in 1980 by William Morrow, Robert Edwards describes how he envisioned the process of in vitro fertilization as early as 1962. "Inject an infertile woman with hormones early in her menstrual cycle, then give a spot of HCG (Human chorionic gonadotropin, the pregnancy hormone released by the uterus when a fertilized egg implants in the uterine lining; it was known at this time to stimulate the maturation of multiple eggs in mouse ovaries.) to cause ovulation, perform a small operation 28 hours later and collect the ripening eggs, place the eggs in a culture fluid, collect the husband's semen and fertilize the egg 'in vitro' (in a glass dish), then replant it in the woman's uterus."

At the time Edwards proposed this idea more than twenty years ago, not very much was known about human fertilization. An American scientist, Gregory Pincus, working twenty-five years before that, had discovered that human eggs extracted from the ovaries would mature outside the body, in a culture medium in the laboratory. Surprisingly his work was unknown to Robert Edwards in 1962.

Working at the National Institute for Medical Research at Mill Hill in England, Edwards saw under his microscope a human egg, twenty-eight hours after it was placed in a culture medium in the laboratory, beginning to mature all by itself. Edwards was ecstatic at this discovery. He was preparing a paper to announce his findings when in the course of his research he learned that Pincus had already made the same discovery. What astonished Edwards was that in twenty-five years, no one had followed up on Pincus' remarkable work. He realized the field of human embryology was wide open. He recognized that there was sufficient evidence to continue his research toward the goal of fertilizing a human egg in vitro.

Three years later, on a November evening in 1965, Edwards—now

* *A Matter of Life,* by Robert Edwards and Patrick Steptoe, copyright © 1980 by Finestride Ltd. & Crownchime Ltd.

working at the Physiological Laboratory in Cambridge—went over to his lab where three human eggs were ripening in a culture medium. His intention was to attempt to fertilize the eggs with his own sperm. "I knew that such an exercise would most probably fail," said Edwards in *A Matter of Life.* "In 1965, it was thought by almost everybody that spermatozoa had to be exposed to the secretions of the uterus or fallopian tubes before they had the capacity to fertilize an egg."

Edwards collected his sperm into a specimen jar, then removed the sperm from the seminal fluid by spinning it in a centrifuge and added it to the eggs in the culture medium. He left the eggs and sperm together overnight. When he came back in the morning, he was astounded. "One spermatozoa had passed through the outer membrane of the egg," said Edwards. "However, it was not a complete fertilization. The sperm and egg had not fused. Even so," said Edwards, "it was enormously encouraging." Unfortunately, it was to be several years before Edwards got that close again to fertilizing an egg in vitro.

As the nature of Edwards' work became known in the scientific community in England, the supply of human eggs he needed to conduct his research began to be increasingly difficult to obtain. Many of his colleagues regarded his work as too controversial; others didn't take it seriously. Edwards began to look for other sources of human eggs. The Johns Hopkins University School of Medicine in Baltimore, Maryland, was one of the few places in the world conducting research with ovarian tissue. Edwards applied for a grant and was awarded one by the Ford Foundation in the summer of 1965 to work for six weeks at Johns Hopkins with Howard and Georgeanna Jones, the husband-and-wife research team in the department of gynecology and obstetrics. In just two weeks at Hopkins, Edwards was able to establish that the ripening process of the human egg, in vitro, took thirty-six hours. But Edwards did not succeed in fertilizing a single egg.

Edwards tried it again in the summer of 1966 at the University of North Carolina at Chapel Hill. This time he modified the technique he had used in 1965 by using sperm which had been exposed in a very complex and elaborate manner to uterine secretions. Still there was no fertilization. Edwards was convinced, though, that this was the way to go —using sperm that had been in contact with the uterus.

It was a year later, while he was browsing through medical journals in the library at Cambridge, that Edwards came across an article written by an obstetrician, Patrick Steptoe, that described just the technique Edwards needed to collect sperm that had been exposed to uterine secretions directly from the fallopian tubes after intercourse. The technique was called a laparoscopy. The author of the article was a gynecologist practicing in a provincial general hospital in Oldham, England, a distance of 165 kilometers from Cambridge.

Laparoscopy, as described in Steptoe's article, was a technique with which, by means of a small incision in the navel, under general anesthesia, the doctor had access to a woman's entire reproductive system. The usual method for gaining access to a woman's reproductive organs at that time was the procedure known as laparotomy, a major surgical intervention requiring a long incision across the abdomen and a lengthy and painful convalescence. Laparotomy was the only accurate method for diagnosing infertility problems that involved the reproductive organs. Steptoe proposed that laparoscopy could now take the place of this painful surgery in diagnosing infertility problems.

The medical profession surprisingly had not rushed to embrace the laparoscopic technique. While his colleagues were dragging their heels, Edwards felt there wasn't a moment to lose. He called Steptoe on the telephone the next day and presented to him the idea of achieving fertilization of a human egg outside the body, with the help of the laparoscopic technique. Edwards expected the usual polite disinterest that greeted any discussion of his work, so he was astonished when, without a moment's hesitation, Steptoe said, "Let's have a try."

The technique of laparoscopy is not new. According to Steptoe in *A Matter of Life*, the forerunner of the laparoscope, a miniature microscope, was the cystoscope, an instrument inserted into the abdomen and used for visualizing the interior of the bladder. An English surgeon used the cystoscope for the purpose of observing the female reproductive organs for the first time in 1925. The cystoscope was perfected as an instrument specifically for the purpose of observing the pelvic organs by a New York gynecologist named Albert Decker in the 1940s. The drawback of Decker's instrument was that it was designed to be inserted through the vagina, between the back of the uterus and the front of the rectum. This was uncomfortable for the patient and incurred the risk of infections.

It was a Parisian gynecologist named Raoul Palmer who became the first to use the instrument by inserting it into the abdominal cavity through an incision in the navel. The procedure required general anesthesia, but did not involve a lengthy convalescence. The patient was able to get up and walk about soon afterward.

Patrick Steptoe heard about Palmer's work in the summer of 1958 at an international medical conference in Montreal. Steptoe had long been

frustrated in his treatment of infertile women by his dependence on laparotomy as his only diagnostic tool. He felt certain that there had to be a
simpler means of observing the pelvic organs. As soon as Steptoe heard
about Palmer's method, he went to Paris and spent several days observing
Palmer's work. He saw that Palmer had fitted Decker's instrument with
an eyepiece at the viewing end and a lens at the other end, thereby
transforming the instrument into a miniature microscope.

Then in 1959, a German gynecologist named Hans Frangenheim,
with the help of German lens manufacturers, refined the instrument now
known as the laparoscope. As soon as the laparoscope became commer-
cially available in Germany, Steptoe bought one and practiced using it on
cadavers in his hospital's mortuary. The biggest obstacle to the efficiency
of the laparoscopic procedure at that time was the light attached to the
laparoscope which enabled doctors to see inside the body. The lamp very
quickly overheated, so that the procedure had to be performed rapidly. "It
was a smash and grab affair," said Steptoe in *A Matter of Life*. Still, it was
a major improvement over the laparotomy.

In 1960, Patrick Steptoe performed his first laparoscopy on a live
patient. He was not able to see the pelvic organs as he should have. His
second attempt was a success. "I was able to see clearly the size, texture,
and color of the whole uterus. I inspected the ligament, ovary, and fallopian tubes as well." Over the next seven years, Steptoe perfected the
procedure in his gynecological practice as a diagnostic tool. He also em-
ployed it in certain operative procedures, such as sterilization by tubal
ligation.

By 1964, the German Frangenheim had come up with the ultimate
refinement in the laparoscope. By employing fiber optics, the transmission
of light over microscopic glass fibers, Frangenheim solved the problem of
lighting the abdominal cavity. The light was constant and there was no
danger of it overheating. Doctors could now take all the time they needed
to work in the pelvic area. And no longer did women have to submit to
the painful laparotomy.

Steptoe, Palmer, and others wrote papers on the efficacy of the
laparoscopic technique, which they presented at the first International
Congress of Laparoscopy in Palermo, Italy, in 1964. Still, it was not widely
practiced. In *A Matter of Life* Steptoe remembers he was working on a
medical textbook on laparoscopy for gynecologists in 1967 when he got
the telephone call from Robert Edwards. "I'm willing to help as much as
possible," he told Edwards. But Robert Edwards never called him back.

Said Edwards, "We were too far away from each other. How could we collaborate at a distance of 165 kilometers?"

It was not until a year later, at a meeting of the Endocrinological and Gynecological Sections of the Royal Society of Medicine in 1968, that Patrick Steptoe and Robert Edwards met and agreed to collaborate on the work that would lead to the birth ten years later of Louise Brown, the first baby conceived outside its mother's womb.

In the decade between their meeting and the birth of Louise Brown, the two men experienced many disappointments, turned down many blind alleys. They started on one track and ended on another. Ironically, their breakthrough occurred when Edwards recognized that his initial premise that sperm had to be exposed to uterine secretions in order to be able to fertilize an egg was incorrect. He found that sperm could be "capacitated"—empowered with the ability to penetrate the egg—by incubating them for several hours in the laboratory. But if Edwards hadn't been convinced of that hypothesis initially, however, he never would have met Steptoe. Steptoe's laparoscopic technique, which he'd originally thought necessary to obtain the sperm, subsequently became the method by which mature eggs could be removed from the ovaries. After this breakthrough, the technique of in vitro fertilization was vastly simplified.

Along the way, technological developments, such as the evolution of fiber optics, aided Steptoe and Edwards' research. So did the discovery by a Cambridge University student of a culture medium called Hams F-10, which allowed mouse embryos to develop; this culture medium was put to use in their research as the culture medium for human embryos.

There were constant challenges to Steptoe and Edwards' work, by the medical authorities who refused to fund their research for ethical reasons, by theologians, and even by their fellow scientists, men of the stature of James Watson, winner of the Nobel prize with Francis Crick for their discovery of the molecular structure of DNA. Among those who supported the in vitro work was Howard Jones and Georgeanna Jones at Johns Hopkins, with whom Edwards had worked in the summer of 1965.

The technique of in vitro fertilization that Steptoe and Edwards developed in 1978 was remarkably simple. There were five steps. The first step was waiting for an egg to mature in the woman's ovary. The second step was the removal of the egg from the woman's ovary just prior to ovulation. Once the egg was removed from the patient's ovary, it was put into a special culture medium in a glass dish in the laboratory and kept in an incubator. The third step was the collection of the man's semen. The semen was then treated in the laboratory to separate the sperm from the seminal fluid, and the sperm was then put into an incubator. The fourth step was fertilization. After incubating for several hours, the man's sperm was put into the dish with the woman's egg, and the dish was put back into the incubator for thirty-six to forty-eight hours. If fertilization occurred, the fifth and final step was the transfer of the fertilized egg, the embryo, to the uterus of the woman.

The first step of the in vitro procedure is the most crucial—getting a mature egg. Whether an egg is fertilized inside or outside a woman's body, the egg must be mature in order for fertilization to take place. Therefore, before an egg can be retrieved from the body for in vitro fertilization, the doctor must be able to determine when the egg is mature.

Steptoe and Edwards accomplished this task by monitoring the levels of certain hormones in the woman's urine, daily, from the beginning of her menstrual cycle. During the twenty-eight-day cycle, a rise in the level of estrogen, the hormone released by the ovaries as the egg matures, around the fourteenth day indicates that the woman is nearing ovulation. This increase in the level of estrogen in the body sends a signal to the pituitary gland to secrete another hormone, called the luteinizing hormone (LH). It is LH which triggers the release of the egg from the ovary.

As the patient got closer to ovulation, Steptoe and Edwards started testing the woman's urine every few hours for the presence of LH. When they detected the presence of LH in the urine, they had good reason to believe the egg was mature. They then had twenty-six hours to retrieve the egg from the ovary. If they waited any longer, the egg would be released into the pelvic cavity, where there would be no possibility of retrieving it.

While this method seems foolproof in theory, it is not so in practice. Every woman does not have the same physiological pattern. Some women have twenty-eight-day cycles, others thirty-three-day cycles. Some ovulate in midcycle, others later or earlier. Therefore, no matter how carefully the maturation of the egg is monitored in each patient, there is always the possibility that the decision to retrieve an egg has been made either too early or too late. In the case of Lesley Brown, Steptoe and Edwards waited twenty-six hours after the onset of her LH surge to retrieve her egg. It proved to be the right time for her.

When the egg is mature, it is time then to retrieve it from the patient's body. This is where Steptoe's laparoscopy comes in. The patient is given a general anesthesia. An incision about an inch long is made in her navel, and the abdominal cavity is filled with carbon dioxide gas for the purpose of lifting the abdominal wall away from the pelvic organs so that the doctors have enough room in there to maneuver. The laparoscope is a long thin instrument that resembles a microscope, an eyepiece at one end and a lens at the other. It is inserted through the incision into the abdominal cavity. By looking through the laparoscope, the doctor can see the ovaries and guide the retrieval process.

If there is indeed a ripe follicle on one of the two ovaries, a second small incision is made below the first for the insertion of the retrieval apparatus. A long hollow needle, which is attached to a plastic test tube, is inserted through this second incision to retrieve the egg inside the follicle. With the needle, the doctor punctures the ripe follicle, and by means of a suction device attached to the needle, he aspirates the egg and the fluid surrounding it, into the test tube. The test tube is taken immediately to the laboratory that adjoins the operating room, and examined under the microscope to confirm that the egg is, in fact, mature. The retrieval procedure lasts about thirty minutes.

While the woman is in the operating room, undergoing laparoscopy, the man provides a semen specimen. He must masturbate into a sterile specimen jar, and get the specimen to the laboratory immediately. There it is washed and spun at a high rate of speed in a centrifuge to separate the sperm from the seminal fluid. Then the sperm are put into a petri dish with the culture medium and placed in an incubator for several hours where they acquire the characteristic that enables them to penetrate an egg. Not all of the sperm in the semen specimen that is provided are used. Many of the obstacles to fertilization that exist in the body have been eliminated in the in vitro process. Therefore, not as many sperm are required.

If the egg that has been retrieved from the woman is mature, it is bathed immediately in the same kind of culture medium in which the sperm are incubating, then put into the petri dish with the sperm. The dish containing the egg and sperm are put into the incubator, which maintains them at normal body temperature until fertilization takes place. Within twelve hours, the first signs of fertilization can usually be seen under the microscope. Cells begin to form. The embryo divides into two cells, then four, then eight. It takes about forty to forty-eight hours for an embryo to reach the eight-cell stage.

When the embryo has reached the eight-cell stage, it is time to transfer the embryo to the woman's uterus. The transfer is a very simple procedure. It takes place in the operating room. The woman is fully awake. She lies on the operating table in the regular gynecological position, on her back, her feet in stirrups. In the lab, the embryo is placed in a long thin cannula with a syringe at the end, which is taken immediately into the operating room. The doctor inserts the loaded cannula through the opening of the cervix into the uterus, and flushes the egg out of the tube into the uterus.

The Steptoe and Edwards technique of in vitro fertilization has remained the basis for all in vitro procedure since 1978. For the rest of 1978, Steptoe and Edwards were the only ones in the world practicing the in vitro procedure. In early 1979, Patrick Steptoe was obligated to retire from the National Health Service, and it would be about a year and a half before he and Edwards would resume their in vitro practice in 1980 with private funds at Bourne Hall in Cambridge. Around the same time, an in vitro program at Monash University in Melbourne, Australia, began treating patients under the direction of Dr. Carl Wood. It was the birth of Louise Brown in 1978, and a chance remark, that led to the opening of the first in vitro clinic in the United States in 1980.

In 1978, Dr. Howard Jones, Jr., a gynecologic surgeon, and his wife, Dr. Georgeanna Seegar Jones, a reproductive endocrinologist, were retiring from the faculty of the Johns Hopkins University School of Medicine in the Department of Obstetrics and Gynecology. They had reached the university's mandatory retirement age of sixty-five. A longtime friend and colleague of the Joneses, Dr. Mason Andrews, who was chairman of the newly established Eastern Virginia Medical School's Department of Obstetrics and Gynecology, in Norfolk, Virginia, invited the Joneses to join his staff and continue their work in treating reproduction problems and infertility.

By pure chance, the Drs. Jones arrived in Norfolk on the very same day in July 1978 that Louise Brown was born in England. When a local newspaper reporter telephoned Dr. Andrews to ask for his comments on the event, Dr. Andrews referred the reporter to the Joneses because of their expertise in this area.

As scientists, as well as doctors, Howard and Georgeanna Jones were not surprised when the birth of Louise Brown was announced. "I knew it was only a matter of time," says Dr. Howard Jones, Jr. He is a tall lean man, with a youthful face, who, when he isn't dressed in surgical greens or lab whites, affects a jaunty bow tie and colorful sports jackets. His face is the kind that inspires immediate trust and invites confidences of the most intimate sort. There could be no one more appropriate for the role he has played in bringing hope to thousands of infertile couples.

"We provided Edwards with the first human eggs of any numbers that he'd had to work with," remembers Dr. Jones. "We were interested in Edwards' idea, but at that time the idea of fertilizing an egg in vitro seemed very theoretical and difficult to accomplish. We didn't have the resources at Johns Hopkins to pursue it ourselves." When Robert Edwards left Johns Hopkins, the work on in vitro was not continued, but the Joneses continued to keep in touch with Edwards through the years, visiting him several times at his laboratory in Cambridge. They expected that there would come a time when the idea would turn out to be practical.

The reporter for the local Norfolk newspaper went out to the Joneses' house that day to interview them. They were in the middle of unpacking boxes and arranging furniture. In the course of the interview, the reporter asked, "Would it be possible to set up an in vitro program in Norfolk?"

"I thought it was a flip question," says Dr. Howard Jones, Jr., "and I thought I was giving her a flip answer. I said, 'Sure, all it would take is money.' I thought that was the end of the matter."

"The truth was," says Dr. Jones, "I did think it was possible. We had the three main requirements: *I* knew about surgery and reproductive matters, Georgeanna was a gynecological endocrinologist, and we happened to bring along with us to EVMS our laboratory personnel from Johns Hopkins."

But that wasn't at all the end of it. The next morning the headline in the Norfolk newspaper read: "Doctor Says All It Takes Is Money." The Joneses hadn't been in their offices five minutes when a telephone call came for Georgeanna Jones. It was a former patient of hers. She had helped the patient conceive after many years of infertility. The woman lived in the Norfolk area and had seen the newspaper headline. "I just happen to have a family foundation," she told Dr. Georgeanna Jones. "How much money do you need?"

Two days later, in the living room of the Joneses' new house, most of the boxes still unpacked, Dr. Mason Andrews, Dr. Howard Jones, Jr., Dr. Georgeanna Jones, and Henry Clay Hofheimer II, the president of the Eastern Virginia Medical School Foundation, which receives funds for the medical school, met with the donor, who still, to this day, prefers to be anonymous. They decided unanimously then and there to go ahead and set up the first in vitro clinic in the United States.

The Eastern Virginia Medical School Vital Initiation of Pregnancy Program began with a modest five thousand dollars. "We didn't need any more than that," said Howard Jones. "We needed seed money first to look into the practicality of setting up the thing. It turned out that an in vitro program is not very expensive. It doesn't require any fancy apparatus, it doesn't need a big capital investment. It requires the same things that any standard hospital has: incubators, microscopes, test tubes . . ."

When the Joneses began investigating the feasibility of an in vitro program in Norfolk in 1978, Robert Edwards and Patrick Steptoe had not yet published a scientific paper explaining their method. "We didn't have the cookbook recipe for in vitro fertilization," said Dr. Jones, "but we had a notion of how it was done." This put the Joneses in the position of having to develop their own technique of in vitro fertilization.

While the Joneses worked on the clinical aspects of the program, Dr. Andrews was working on the administrative arrangements. The in vitro program would be organized as part of the Department of Obstetrics and Gynecology and like all the EVMS faculties, would use the laboratory and operating facilities of Norfolk General Hospital. Any hospital is required by federal regulation to apply to the Health Services Administration for a Certificate of Need when a new service is projected. This regulation was designed to prevent duplication of expensive medical services in the same vicinity. No one connected with the EVMS in vitro program anticipated there would be any problem obtaining the necessary certification because the service they were offering was unique in the entire United States.

Dr. Howard Jones, Jr. and Dr. Georgeanna Jones were traveling in Europe when the HSA held public hearings on the medical school's application in the late summer of 1979. To everyone's surprise, a vociferous and well-organized Right to Life group turned up to protest the awarding of the certification. Even the HSA was caught off guard. The agency had not scheduled enough time to hear the number of people who wanted to speak, so the hearing was rescheduled for October 31, 1979. "We hadn't even picked up our first test tube," says Dr. Howard Jones, Jr., "and a whole year had gone by."

When the second hearing was held, the Joneses were prepared. They, as well as the Right-to-Lifers, had martialed an army of prominent people to speak on their behalf. The hearing lasted from two in the afternoon until eight that night. The battle was heated and acrimonious. The national press picked up the story and the Joneses were all over the television evening news programs that night. "Ironically," says Dr. Howard Jones, Jr., "it was by virtue of this publicity that the in vitro program at EVMS became known. It put us in a fish bowl right away. We couldn't afford not to be successful."

The Certificate of Need was eventually granted to the Norfolk General Hospital by the Virginia Health Commissioner in December 1979.

Before the clinic started operation, Dr. Howard Jones, Jr., asked for a three-year commitment from the medical school commissioners and hospital trustees, to get the VIP Program off the ground. "We needed at least that much time to produce results," he says. "The British had been at it for over fifteen years before they succeeded. The Australians had already been working at it for about seven years without a pregnancy." The Joneses were given unanimous approval of their request and directed to proceed. In March 1980, Dr. Howard Jones, Jr., and Dr. Georgeanna Jones began preliminary clinical trials.

The status of in vitro fertilization when the Joneses launched the VIP Program had not changed much since the birth of Louise Brown. There had been only two more births by in vitro fertilization in a year and a half. The third in vitro baby was born in Melbourne, Australia, in 1980.

The technique used by Dr. Howard Jones, Jr., and Dr. Georgeanna Jones in their preliminary trials was based on the English method. The Joneses consulted with Steptoe and Edwards before they began. "Their advice to us," says Dr. Howard Jones, "was to follow the woman's natural menstrual cycle and retrieve the mature egg just prior to ovulation. They stressed that it was absolutely imperative to get the egg to the sperm within ninety seconds after it had been recovered from the ovary."

For the duration of 1980, the Joneses followed Steptoe and Edwards' advice. They selected their first patients from a pool of nearly six thousand applicants. The criteria for selection in the initial phase was that a patient had to be under thirty-five years of age, and that she have no fallopian tubes at all. Women who fit this category were those who had had both fallopian tubes removed as a result of one or more ectopic pregnancies.

An ectopic pregnancy is a pregnancy in which the developing embryo attaches itself to the wall of the fallopian tube instead of passing into the uterus and implanting there. The fallopian tube is damaged beyond repair and the life of the mother threatened if the situation is not detected, and the embryo aborted. The reason why the Joneses specified that their patients have no fallopian tubes was that, if pregnancy were achieved, there would be no doubt whatsoever that it had been achieved in vitro. If pregnancy resulted in a patient in whom one tube, or even part of a tube remained, or the fallopian tubes were diagnosed as obstructed, there would always be a question of doubt. The pregnancy might have been achieved normally, in vivo.

By the end of 1980, the Joneses had treated forty-one patients, following the woman's natural menstrual cycle, and had not achieved a single pregnancy. "The Steptoe and Edwards method clearly wasn't working for us," says Dr. Howard Jones, Jr. Dr. Jones consulted by telephone with Dr. Carl Wood, director of the Australian in vitro program, and found out that his group was also having difficulty achieving a pregnancy using the natural cycle.

Around Christmastime 1980, the Joneses were reevaluating their technique, when Dr. Wood called to tell them that his team was using a new technique. They were giving their in vitro patients a fertility drug called clomiphene. Clomiphene is a drug that is used in patients with hormonal deficiencies to stimulate the ovaries to produce more than one egg during the menstrual cycle. "Steptoe and Edwards had experimented with the stimulated cycle for several years before the birth of Louise Brown," says Dr. Jones, "but it hadn't worked for them." The Joneses considered trying the Australian approach.

Dr. Georgeanna Jones, however, was against using clomiphene. She comes from the same long, lean Chesapeake Bay stock as her husband. In surgical greens, the only way to tell the Joneses apart is by the nose. Howard has a beak nose; Georgeanna has an aristocratic nose. Where Howard is jovial, Georgeanna is all business. Howard is the administrator, the public relations director, and the inspiration behind the EVMS VIP Program; Georgeanna is the scientist, the theoretician, and the practitioner of the EVMS in vitro technique.

Dr. Georgeanna Jones had been working for many years in her private gynecological practice in Baltimore with women whose infertility was caused by a failure to ovulate due to hormonal deficiencies. In case after case, she had been successful in stimulating ovulation and achieving pregnancy in these women by administering the hormone HMG, human menopausal gonadotropin. HMG is made up of two elements—FSH, follicle stimulating hormone, and LH, luteinizing hormone, (both produced by the pituitary gland) in a ratio of one to one.

HMG and clomiphene perform the same function. They both stimulate the ovaries to produce more than one egg on a given cycle; they have been known to produce as many as twenty eggs in one cycle. The mechanism by which these two drugs achieve follicle growth, however, is different. HMG acts directly on the ovaries to stimulate follicle growth. Clomiphene acts on the pituitary gland to produce FSH and LH, which then stimulate the ovaries to grow follicles. HMG is a natural substance, found in the body. Clomiphene is an artificial substance. "I chose HMG to work with in my gynecology practice," says Dr. Georgeanna Jones, "because it is a natural hormone. We knew a normal egg survived it, but we didn't know about the effects of clomiphene."

Based on her experience with HMG, Dr. Georgeanna Jones suggested that on their next round of in vitro patients, they use HMG to stimulate the ovaries to mature multiple eggs. The more eggs that were available, the greater the chances were that one or more of them would be mature when the laparoscopic retrieval was performed. The more mature eggs that could be retrieved, the greater the chances were that one or more of them would fertilize. "What we would be doing," explains Dr. Georgeanna Jones, "was taking normally ovulating patients, and trying to make them do something abnormal, produce more than one egg. If we could do it in abnormal, nonovulating patients, I didn't see why we couldn't do it in normal ovulatory patients." The Joneses went to Serono Laboratories for their HMG, which is marketed under the trade name Pergonal.

Therefore, going against the advice of Steptoe and Edwards to follow a woman's natural menstrual cycle, the Joneses initiated the technique of the hormone stimulated cycle in January 1981. The dosage of HMG given to the patients was determined on the basis of Dr. Georgeanna Jones's experience. "The usual theory about administering medicine," she explains, "is to use as little as possible and as much as necessary, but that's not the most efficient way to use gonadotropins. It's best to start with the highest dosage necessary, then *reduce.*" Dr. Jones started to see results immediately. "We were getting as many as three and four ripe follicles in our patients," she says. The policy of the EVMS VIP Program at that time was to retrieve all of the eggs, and attempt to fertilize as many of them as were mature.

The Joneses also discarded Edwards' advice that there must be no more than ninety seconds between the time the egg is retrieved and united with the sperm. Following the practice of Dr. Wood and the Melbourne group, the Joneses decided to preincubate the eggs after their retrieval for at least eight hours prior to insemination. "The difference was extraordinary," says Dr. Howard Jones, Jr. "The percentage of eggs that fertilized increased enormously when we preincubated them before uniting them with the sperm. It isn't surprising when you stop to think about it. In the normal process of fertilization, the human egg is mature when it is released from the ovary. In the in vitro procedure, we are retrieving the egg from the ovary, just prior to ovulation. Therefore, just sitting in an armchair and thinking about it, it makes sense that the egg isn't as ripe when we retrieve it as it would be when it is released from the ovary and enters the fallopian tubes. The preincubation fills in that gap of time, and allows the egg to reach its full maturity before it meets the sperm."

While the Joneses were developing the hormone stimulation and egg retrieval techniques for the EVMS VIP Program, embryologist Lucinda Veeck was working on the laboratory methods. Mrs. Veeck developed methods of monitoring the eggs after retrieval, incubating the eggs, preparing the sperm, and overseeing the fertilization. Mrs. Veeck's most significant contribution was her success in maturing eggs that were retrieved from the ovaries in an immature condition. "By preincubating immature eggs for up to thirty-six hours, we were able to mature them," says Mrs. Veeck. As a result, a follicle does not have to be fully mature in order to be harvested. This capacity to mature immature eggs in the incubator increases still more the number of eggs that can be retrieved from the ovary, thereby enhancing the chances that fertilization will occur.

The Joneses were treating their first thirty-one patients with the new technique of the stimulated cycle when Dr. Rachel Schachter wrote to Dr. Howard Jones, Jr., on behalf of Nan and Todd Tilton in March 1981. The criteria by which candidates were chosen then were the following:

1. Infertility due to a condition not amenable to conventional therapy. Such conditions include: tubal disease, sperm abnormalities, untreatable cervical factors, and "normal" infertile couples (couples in whom the cause of infertility is unexplained).

2. Preference will be given to patients who have had both fallopian tubes removed (bilateral salpingectomies).

3. Patients preferably should be under the age of thirty-five, but in no case over the age of forty.

4. Patients should have at least one ovary available for laparoscopy.

5. There must be no evidence of serious menstrual irregularities.

6. Patients must have a normal uterus.

The VIP Program emphasized that the in vitro procedure is not a solution for infertility in the male due to azospermia (no sperm). A woman must have at least one ovary and a uterus for in vitro fertilization to be attempted.

When Dr. Schachter's referral letter arrived, it could have gone unnoticed among the six thousand other letters the Joneses had received requesting treatment by in vitro fertilization. But many of those potential patients had turned out to be medically unqualified for the in vitro procedure. Some applicants could not be found; they had moved and left no forwarding addresses. Some couples had gotten divorced, and others had conceived on their own or adopted a child. "Many patients, when they heard we hadn't had any pregnancies yet, decided not to come," says Dr. Howard Jones, Jr. "It wasn't as easy as we thought it was going to be to find patients."

So when the Tiltons' referral arrived, there was not a long list of patients scheduled for treatment. Still, the Tiltons might have been rejected. "At that point," said Dr. Jones, "we weren't treating patients with bilateral infertility problems. We hadn't yet addressed the problem of low sperm counts." But the Joneses had decided they would begin to accept oligospermic patients when Dr. Schachter's letter arrived. "See what I mean?" says Todd. "God *was* watching over us. How else would you explain that we always happened to be doing the right thing at the right time?"

For Nan Tilton, the last few weeks of March could not go fast enough. Would Dr. Schachter call her when she got a letter? Should Nan call her? Nan did, between classes at the phone booth out by the maintenance shed. "I'll call you," Dr. Schachter told her.

Five weeks later, on April 15, Nan had her answer. Dr. Schachter read the letter to her over the telephone. Nan has a copy of the letter in a scrapbook, with one sentence underlined in red ink. "It is unlikely that we will be successful in achieving a pregnancy," wrote Dr. Howard Jones, Jr., "but we could give it a try." As Nan listened, the nursery school children burst out of the door into the playground. One little boy struggled to reach the first step on the slide and fell. Nan swallowed, watching him, unable to speak. Dr. Jones's letter continued. "In the Tiltons' case, there is a bilateral problem. We feel that such patients are candidates for in vitro, provided that at least 1 million sperm can be obtained. If Mr. and Mrs. Tilton are interested, they need to make a preliminary appointment for review of their situation."

"Do you realize what this meant?" Nan whispers. "Todd and I weren't being offered a long shot to have someone else's baby. Dr. Jones was offering us the chance to have *our very own baby, Todd's and mine.* Not a single one of our doctors had ever given us this hope."

The very same day that Nan Tilton received her letter from the Eastern Virginia Medical School VIP Program, Judy Carr from Westminster, Massachusetts, the thirteenth patient to be treated by the Norfolk clinic with the new technique of the stimulated cycle, was wheeled into the operating room for her egg retrieval. Two eggs, "normal preovulatory oocytes" is the technical term, were aspirated from two follicles on Mrs. Carr's ovaries by the laparoscopic technique and put into the incubator. Six hours later, her husband Roger Carr's sperm were added to the petri dish with the eggs. About twenty-two hours later, the cells had begun to divide. Fertilization had taken place in both eggs. When the fertilized eggs, two human embryos, reached the eight-cell stage, they were both transferred to the uterus of Judy Carr. It would be ten days before Dr. Howard Jones, Jr., and Dr. Georgeanna Jones and the EVMS in vitro team knew for certain that they had achieved the first in vitro pregnancy in the United States.

5

The Screening

At the end of April 1981, the application forms from the Vital Initiation of Pregnancy Program at Eastern Virginia Medical School arrived at Dr. Schachter's office. Nan went over to pick it up. "There were pages and pages of information about the in vitro procedure, and questionnaires that had to be filled out," says Nan. "I took everything home and spread it all out on the dining room table and read every word on every page. I couldn't get enough of those words. I devoured them."

Included in the packet of information was a list of qualifications for acceptance, an explanation of the in vitro process, a questionnaire for Todd as part of the special program for husbands with low sperm counts, a schedule and description of the treatment and procedures involved, and a list of costs.

The cost of the entire in vitro procedure was divided into two parts. The first part was a preliminary visit, which cost $500, and the in vitro attempt, which cost $3,500. These costs did not include food and lodging for a couple's preliminary visit to Norfolk, nor for the three-week stay required for the in vitro attempt; nor did they include the cost of any preliminary surgical procedures that might be necessary to prepare the patient for the in vitro procedure. "We were talking about something like $8,000," says Todd. "And insurance companies didn't cover all the cost because in vitro fertilization was regarded as an experimental procedure."

The application made it clear that a patient should be prepared to try in vitro fertilization at least three times. Therefore a minimum of $11,000 could be required for medical costs alone. The medical cost in 1985, four years later, for one in vitro trial is $4,833.

Nan started saving her paychecks to set aside the $11,000 in a separate bank account. "We were lucky," says Nan. "We could afford it. One woman I heard about lived on hot dogs for a year to be able to pay for it. Another couple sold everything they had and came to Norfolk in a trailer. Other people mortgaged their houses."

The VIP application made it clear that before any appointment would be set up, applicants were to fill out all the questionnaires and make sure that the clinic received a complete set of medical records, including hysterosalpingograms and copies of doctors' notes on operations performed prior to the in vitro attempt, including laparoscopies.

The application continued: "If on the basis of information supplied by this questionnaire and your gynecologist it seems reasonable to pursue the matter, it will be necessary for you to make a preliminary visit to Norfolk in order to make further arrangements. An andrology survey (a detailed sperm analysis) is part of this visit. After the Preliminary Consultation, depending on the situation, one of several alternatives may then be pursued:

1. It may seem desirable to proceed further.

2. Additional studies or procedures may be necessary before a final judgement can be made about the feasibility of the VIP Program for you.

3. A screening diagnostic laparoscopy may prove necessary to evaluate the suitability of your pelvic structure for admission to the program. This can usually be scheduled for a day or two after the preliminary consultation . . . You are not admitted to the VIP Program until your suitability has been determined by the screening diagnostic laparoscopy."

The application brochure concluded with a realistic assessment of the status of in vitro fertilization. "It is important," stated the brochure, "that those who embark on this program understand that the chance of success in any one fertilization attempt is quite small. Normal fertile couples who become pregnant in the natural way achieve a pregnancy which results in a term delivery after an average exposure of three months. This means that some couples in normal circumstances become pregnant after one exposure, others require up to several months or a year. The *average number of exposures is three.* It is, of course, very unlikely that the VIP Program will be able to improve on the biological circumstances which make an average of three exposures necessary."

Nan carefully filled out the application and questionnaire. Within a week she had contacted every single one of the doctors who had treated her and Todd for their infertility problems in the past three years—the urologist who identified Todd's infertility problem: low sperm count; Dr.

Richard Amelar, who performed bilateral varicocele surgery on Todd to reverse his infertility, without success; Dr. Rachel Schachter, who attempted artificial insemination three times on Nan Tilton without success, and as a result made a preliminary diagnosis of Nan's infertility problem: blocked fallopian tubes. Dr. Philip Rice, who performed the hysterosalpingogram, lent evidence to this diagnosis of Nan's infertility problem, and Dr. William Lipkin confirmed it with a diagnostic laparoscopy. Dr. Lipkin's recommendation that Nan have two major surgeries to open up the ends of her fallopian tubes, giving her a 10 percent chance of becoming pregnant, was refused by the Tiltons.

The only doctor the Tiltons did not contact was Dr. Ernest Samuelson, the first infertility specialist they had consulted in 1978. If the Tiltons had found out three years earlier the exact nature of their infertility problems, would they have considered in vitro fertilization? "After Louise Brown was born, I would have gone to England right away to Steptoe and Edwards," says Nan. But Nan and Todd would have put their hope in in vitro fertilization too early, when it was still a dream for the future.

Three years later, in 1981, when Nan sent off her application to Norfolk, in vitro fertilization was still a dream, but it was exactly the right moment, the moment when in vitro fertilization was about to become a reality of modern life. "I keep saying," says Todd, "there's been a hand guiding us, making sure we ended up right where we did, when we did. We had the experience behind us and the timing was right, so that we could put everything we had into making in vitro fertilization work for us."

Nan completed the application in the first week of May, and mailed it off to Norfolk. A week later, on May 12, 1981, the New York *Times* reported the first pregnancy by in vitro fertilization had been achieved at the Eastern Virginia Medical School in Norfolk, Virginia, under the direction of Dr. Howard Jones, Jr. The woman was not identified, but in fact it was Judy Carr.

Judy Carr and her husband, Roger Carr, from Westminster, Massachusetts, came to the Norfolk clinic in January 1981. They had been trying since 1977 to have children. She was twenty-eight, he was thirty. They had been married for several years. Judy waited until she got her college degree to try and get pregnant. She became pregnant the summer after she graduated, right on schedule. Two months later she was rushed to the hospital with severe cramps. Her doctor discovered an ectopic pregnancy. Instead of developing in the uterus, the embryo had implanted in her right fallopian tube and was developing there. The tube had ruptured and caused internal bleeding, which threatened her life. The fallopian tube had to be removed, along with the embryo. Her left fallopian tube was undamaged and she was told she still had a chance of becoming pregnant and carrying a baby to term.

The next summer Judy Carr got pregnant again. This pregnancy too turned out to be an ectopic pregnancy. This time, however, it was discovered in time to remove the embryo from the tube before it ruptured. Judy and Roger Carr tried again in September 1980. After two months, Judy Carr went to the hospital with her third ectopic pregnancy. Her remaining fallopian tube was removed. After the operation, her doctor told her that she and her husband had no possibility now of conceiving their own child. In proposing alternatives, he mentioned he had seen articles in the newspaper about a program in Norfolk, Virginia, that was taking women without fallopian tubes for in vitro fertilization. Judy and Roger Carr did not waste any time. They decided to pursue two things at once—adoption and in vitro fertilization.

The Carrs had their first appointment at EVMS's VIP Program in January 1981. Dr. Jairo Garcia, an obstetrician/gynecologist on the Norfolk in vitro team, performed a diagnostic laparoscopy on Judy Carr to determine the condition of her uterus and ovaries, and to find out if any adhesions had grown since her tubes had been removed. The laparoscopy revealed that one of Judy's ovaries was 90 percent accessible for egg retrieval, but the other was only 60 percent accessible. But because she fit the program's requirement that patients have no fallopian tubes, Judy Carr was accepted as a candidate for in vitro fertilization.

On April 8, Judy Carr began her treatment with daily injections of Pergonal to increase the number of eggs the ovaries produced. On April 15, she was taken into the operating room for her egg retrieval. Dr. Jones performed the laparoscopy. "We found that two follicles had developed. We aspirated two eggs; one was a perfect preovulatory oocyte, the other was immature." A few hours later, Roger Carr was requested to deliver a semen specimen. Afterward Judy and Roger Carr left the hospital.

The preovulatory egg was put into an incubator in the lab and was allowed to develop for six hours. At the end of six hours, Roger Carr's sperm was put into the glass dish that held the egg. Forty-eight hours later, the egg had fertilized and become an eight-celled embryo. It was time now for the embryo to be transferred to Judy Carr's uterus. The transfer took place on April 17. The procedure lasted only a few minutes. Judy Carr had to lie still on her stomach for four hours afterward, then she and her husband went back to their hotel.

Judy Carr stayed in Norfolk for the next two weeks. The in vitro team monitored her blood every other day and watched the levels of estrogen rise. They suspected she might be pregnant, but they could not be certain until ten days had passed. Two weeks went by and Judy Carr did not get her period. On April 27, Judy Carr's pregnancy test was positive. It was only then that Judy and Roger Carr learned that theirs was the first in vitro pregnancy achieved at the Norfolk clinic, and the first in the United States.

Nan Tilton read and clipped every newspaper article about Judy Carr's pregnancy that she could get her hands on and put them in a scrapbook. She tape recorded every television report. The difference, though, in the Carrs' infertility situation and the Tiltons' was significant. "It was this sperm thing that made our situation so iffy," says Nan. Nan read and reread the paragraph in Silber's book, *How to Get Pregnant,* that explained why in vitro fertilization was a potential solution for couples with low sperm counts. Nan went back to the library and made photo copies of all the news stories surrounding the birth of Louise Brown in England in 1978. "I added a picture of Lesley Brown and her baby to my scrapbook," says Nan. "I looked at that picture every night and every morning, and thought, She did it. It can work. It can work for us." And all day long, over and over, like a refrain, Nan was sending messages to Norfolk, Please take us, please take us, please . . .

After the Memorial Day holiday, the Tiltons received their answer. The letter from Dr. Jairo Garcia read, "I have reviewed your records. . . . We have a bilateral problem which we will have to evaluate very carefully. . . . It will be necessary that you come to Norfolk for a preliminary visit. Mr. Tilton should submit a semen specimen that will be evaluated in our Andrology Lab. Mrs. Tilton needs to have another diagnostic laparoscopy to see how many adhesions there are, and if the ovaries are available for the aspiration of the follicles in the near future. If you are interested, contact Mrs. Linda Lynch, our administrative assistant, and make the necessary arrangements."

"Were we interested?" asked Nan. "I called Linda Lynch on the telephone that instant to schedule our appointment." It was the beginning of June. Nan would have to wait at least two more weeks until school was out. Todd had been saving his vacation for summer sailing trips, so he still had all his vacation days to use. The appointment was to be scheduled for as soon after the woman's menstrual period as possible. Nan made the appointment for July 13, 1981, at 1:00 P.M.

A week later a letter arrived, confirming the date and giving instructions. Todd would be required to provide a semen specimen the day they arrived. He and Nan were to abstain from sexual intercourse for three to five days prior to the visit so that there would be a representative sample of sperm. A container and instructions for the collection of the sperm were enclosed. It was to be done no sooner than thirty minutes before the Tiltons came to the office at one o'clock. Nan's screening diagnostic laparoscopy would be done the following day, Tuesday, July 14, at twelve.

The total cost of these procedures in 1981 was $1,350. The entire amount had to be paid by check or cash at the time of the visit. The amount was broken down into the following charges:

Initial Visit (Administrative Charge)	$ 100.00
Andrology Survey (Semen Analysis)	150.00
Includes repeat studies if necessary	
Laparoscopy (professional fee)	300.00
Hospital Deposit	800.00
	$ 1,350.00

In 1985, the same procedures cost $1,500.00.

By the end of July 1981, the EVMS VIP Program had completed its first cycle of patients treated with the stimulated ovulation technique. "We sat down and analyzed the results," says Dr. Georgeanna Jones. "We had twelve patient transfers, and two pregnancies in that group. So we decided to continue with the stimulated cycle on our next group of patients."

On the morning of July 13, Todd Tilton's parents drove Nan and Todd to LaGuardia Airport for their flight to Norfolk. "We told both of our families this time what we were doing," says Nan, "but no one else knew, not then." Their families were optimistic about the outcome, as were Nan and Todd. It was a short airplane flight, barely two hours. At the Norfolk airport, Nan and Todd rented a car and drove from the outskirts of Norfolk to the city proper and the Omni Hotel.

The Omni Hotel had been recommended to Nan by the clinic's administrative assistant, Linda Lynch. The Omni provided reduced rates for VIP Program patients. At that time, a room cost thirty-five dollars a night, half the usual rate. Now it is up to fifty dollars, but there are other hotels in the area which offer reduced rates for VIP patients, others with more reasonable rates, such as the Holiday Inn at Waterside and the Madison Hotel. In the cheaper range are rooms for eight dollars a night at the Central Baptist Church's Caring Center. But what these accommodations lack is a significant element of the in vitro process—the companionship and support of other in vitro patients. A list of accommodations in low, moderate, and expensive price ranges is included in the packet of information the Norfolk clinic sends to prospective patients.

The Omni Hotel turned out to be in the area of Norfolk known as Waterside, which is right on the Norfolk harbor, one of the biggest ports in the eastern United States. Nan and Todd pulled up into the driveway and the porter, wearing a pith helmet, khaki shirt and bermuda shorts, knee socks and oxfords, ran to open the car door. He offered his arm to Nan to help her out of the car, unloaded the suitcases from the trunk, then took the keys from Todd to park the car.

Nan and Todd went in the rather unassuming entrance to find themselves in a grandiose lobby more befitting a museum than a hotel. Marble floors stretched as far as the eye could see to a cocktail lounge sunken several steps below, and a wall of windows looking out on the harbor. Along one side of the lobby was the hotel desk; along the other, deep sofas and arm chairs upholstered in green and beige prints were arranged to create discreet conversation areas. There was not a soul to be seen in the lobby when Nan and Todd arrived.

The porter showed them to their room. It was at the back of the hotel, overlooking the swimming pool and the harbor. The room was disappointing in contrast to the lobby; it was decorated in beige and mustard and smelled slightly musty. It was by then almost noon. Nan and Todd had time for a quick bite in the hotel coffee shop, twice as expensive as they had imagined. "We didn't go there too often after that," says Nan. Then they went back to the room so that Todd could produce his semen specimen. It didn't take long. "I was used to it by this time," says Todd.

Nan changed her clothes. She put on a navy blue linen skirt and short, waist-length red jacket. Her hair hung just to her shoulders. She looked blond and tan from weekends on the sailboat. She put on a little more blue eye shadow to make her eyes look bluer, and she was ready. She looked at Todd in his navy blue suit. He was wearing one of his pink shirts with the monogram on the pocket. Todd always looked great. They really made a very elegant couple. Nan was satisfied. "I wanted them to *like* us," says Nan. "They couldn't turn us away if they liked us." Todd went out to the parking lot for the car.

Following the directions given to them by Linda Lynch, Nan and

Todd drove to Norfolk General Hospital and found Medical Tower. Medical Tower is a professional building where many doctors affiliated with the hospital have their offices. Nan and Todd took the elevator to the sixth floor. Room 603 was just to the right of the elevator. The VIP offices were later moved to Room 304. "Obstetrics/Gynecology" read the sign on the door. Nan paused a moment to take a deep breath. She was so excited, she could hardly breathe. "Do I look all right?" she whispered to Todd. "Fine," he said. He pushed open the door.

Inside was a typical doctor's waiting room—deep pile orange carpets, sofas and chairs upholstered in tan and orange arranged in two separate seating areas with coffee tables full of current magazines. Heavy ginger jar lamps cast a warm glow over the room; it could have been any time of day or night and the room would have looked the same. Two doors, one at either end of the room, undoubtedly led to the examining rooms and offices.

There were no other patients waiting, nor was there a sign of a receptionist. Suddenly a frosted glass panel in the wall to the left of the door opened. A woman put her head out. "Hello," she said. "Todd and Nan Tilton," said Todd. "We have an appointment with Dr. Garcia. Meanwhile, what do I do with this?" Todd held out his semen specimen. "I'll take it," she said. "I'm Linda Lynch." "Oh, hi," said Nan. "Thank you so much for your directions. We didn't have any trouble getting here." "I'm glad to meet you finally," said Linda, "after all our telephone conversations. Please have a seat and Dr. Garcia will be right with you."

Nan sat down on the edge of a chair and Todd went exploring. At the end of the room was a bulletin board. "All VIP patients, please keep basal temperature charts," he read. Nan looked anxiously toward the doors, first one, then the other. "Listen to this, Nan," said Todd, reading. "Success begins with a fellow's will, it's all in the state of mind . . . Sooner or later the man who wins is the man who thinks he can . . . I guess we came to the right place," said Todd. One of the doors opened then and Linda Lynch came out. "You can go in now," she said, and they followed her down a short corridor to Dr. Garcia's office.

Dr. Jairo Garcia is one of several obstetrician/gynecologists on the EVMS in vitro team. He was born in Colombia, South America. He came to the United States in 1974, as a fellow at Johns Hopkins in the Department of Obstetrics and Gynecology under Dr. Howard Jones, Jr. When the Joneses retired, Dr. Garcia returned to his native Colombia to start his own infertility practice. When Howard Jones was certain the EVMS in vitro program would be a reality, he knew the one man he wanted for his staff was Jairo Garcia. Dr. Garcia did not hesitate. He came back to the U.S. with his wife and three children in 1979 and has worked with the Joneses at Norfolk from the very beginning.

A handsome, dark-haired man, with a face ravaged by the consequences of the empathy that emanates involuntarily from his presence, came from behind his desk to shake their hands. "It is nice to meet you," he said formally in a quiet voice. "Please sit down." It was the rhythm of his phrases, more than his pronunciation, that revealed his foreign origins. It compelled the listener to listen. "The next two days will be critical in determining whether you will be accepted into the VIP Program," he said. He explained what would happen in those two days during the preliminary visit.

On the first day, the doctor would study the couple's medical history, then do a complete physical exam of the wife. The husband's semen would be sent to the laboratory for a routine semen analysis, his sperm checked for motility, quality, and volume. On the second day, the wife would be given a screening laparoscopy at Norfolk General Hospital. Under general anesthesia, Dr. Garcia would perform a laparoscopy to look at the ovaries and to determine if they were available for the retrieval of eggs by laparoscope. "The screening laparoscopy is a key procedure because it indicates the direction we will take in the future," explained Dr. Garcia.

Dr. Garcia told them that there are several conditions that can be revealed by this laparoscopy. One possibility is that the ovaries are free and unhampered, and the fallopian tubes are damaged beyond repair or absent completely. In this case, the patient is ready for in vitro fertilization and may set up an appointment to come back to Norfolk for an in vitro fertilization attempt. The appointment must be scheduled for at least six weeks after the screening laparoscopy takes place. This six-week period gives the body time to eliminate the effects of the anesthesia administered during the laparoscopy.

Another condition which can be observed during laparoscopy is a very severe scarring of the ovaries and fallopian tubes, which obscures the ovaries completely. "In the past," says Dr. Garcia, "we rejected those patients for in vitro fertilization. Now we are working on a new technique to aspirate the eggs, not by laparoscopy, but with the guidance of ultrasound. Instead of taking the patient to the operating room and putting her under anesthesia, we can, in the examining room, locate the follicle by ultrasound and insert a needle through the bladder, into the abdominal cavity, and aspirate the follicle this way. The patients we rejected in the past who had this condition will be able to come back now for an in vitro attempt."

A third condition revealed by laparoscopy is that some degree of scarring on the ovaries does exist, but they are potentially accessible. In this case, the patient is admitted to the VIP Program, but with the understanding that there might be some problems in retrieving all of the eggs that develop because they might be located in a part of the ovaries that is not accessible. "This is not an ideal situation," says Dr. Garcia, "but we can work with it, provided a good part of the ovary is available."

In other cases, adhesions cover the ovaries in such a way that another surgery is indicated. The purpose of this surgery is to remove the scar tissue, and the damaged fallopian tubes, then move the ovaries close to the uterus, and suspend the uterus. In this way, the patient's ovaries can be made available to the laparoscope. These patients come to Norfolk for the surgery, then are sent home. Three months later, they may come back for their in vitro attempt.

Finally, there are patients in whom one ovary is covered by adhesions and the other ovary is free and available. By using ultrasound, the doctors can determine when follicles are developing on the good ovary and the in vitro attempt can be made.

As Nan Tilton listened to Dr. Garcia, she felt any doubts she might have had about in vitro fertilization disappearing. "I would have done anything this man told me to do," says Nan. "I trusted him completely." But Todd wanted to know what the chances of success were. Dr. Garcia smiled. "We are awaiting news of our second pregnancy this very day." Nan and Todd looked at each other. "We had no idea," says Nan. "One pregnancy . . . that was all."

Nan was surprised to discover that somehow it didn't make any difference. "I realized I didn't care what the odds were," says Nan. "It was a chance, the only chance we had, for Todd and me to have our very own baby. I knew instinctively that Dr. Garcia was going to work as hard as he possibly could to make me pregnant . . . if only he would take us." There Nan and Todd Tilton were, dressed up in their Sunday School best, smiling, being charming, begging Dr. Garcia to like them. But it wasn't up to Dr. Garcia. It depended on Nan and Todd, on the status of Todd's sperm and the accessibility of Nan's ovaries.

After Nan and Todd's appointment with Dr. Garcia, they had nothing to do but wait until Nan's screening laparoscopy the next day. They went back to the hotel. From the window of their room, they looked down on the swimming pool. There were a few families, but what was immediately apparent was that there was a group of women who had pulled their lounge chairs together to be close to each other. Were they in vitro patients? How Nan longed to be one of them.

Nan and Todd had dinner in the hotel dining room that night. Nan was not to eat or drink anything after midnight. After dinner they went to bed. They arrived at the hospital the next morning at seven-thirty. Nan was taken into a room, where she took off her clothes and put on a hospital gown. Todd was permitted to come in and wait with her until the surgery. Anesthesia was not administered until the last minute, when the patient was lying on the operating table. It was a precaution the doctors took, both in screening laparoscopies and in in vitro laparoscopies. In the event that the doctors should find a ripened follicle on the ovary during the screening laparoscopy, it could be aspirated right then for an in vitro fertilization attempt. Since the effects of anesthesia on maturing eggs was still unknown, the less time the egg was exposed to the anesthesia, the better.

Nan was nervous. "I had to keep going to the bathroom," she says. Then the nurse came in and walked Nan down the hall to the operating room. In the operating room, two nurses helped Nan get up onto the table, put in an IV, and draped her with sterile cloths. They put leg warmers on her legs, "to keep the circulation going," explained the nurse. Nan already felt cold. "I started trembling and couldn't stop myself," says Nan. The nurse assured her this was a common reaction. Finally the nurses tipped the operating table to a 45-degree angle so that Nan's head was down and her legs up in the air, "This way the intestines and other organs fall away from the ovaries and uterus," Dr. Garcia explained.

Dr. Garcia was unrecognizable in his surgical mask. It was his voice that reassured Nan. He told her what he was going to do. "I worried about the anesthetic," says Nan. "I didn't want to get sick again the way I did after Dr. Lipkin's laparoscopy." The anesthesiologist said he'd give her less then. Everything was ready. The anesthesiologist began the drip into her veins.

Nan woke up thirty minutes later in the recovery room. Todd was there next to her bed. She was glad to discover she felt only slightly sick this time. She remained in the recovery room for an hour until she was fully awake and her vital signs were stable, then she got dressed and Todd took her back to the hotel.

At seven-thirty the next morning, Nan and Todd went over to Medical Tower to find out the results of their tests. They met Dr. Garcia in the lobby and rode up with him in the elevator. "He was so nice," says Todd.

"We were to find out that Dr. Garcia treated all of his patients as though they were very special to him." Nan tried to read in Dr. Garcia's expression the verdict on their case. "He was so warm, such a gentle man," says Nan. "I had the feeling that everything was going to be all right." The Tiltons followed Dr. Garcia into his office.

Dr. Garcia had the Tiltons' medical records spread out on the desk in front of him. "Let me explain the situation," he said. "Mr. Tilton has a sperm count of over 1 million. This is very good, but we must be sure it stays over 1 million. We need that many to be able to concentrate and prepare the sperm so that a minimum of 50,000 normal-appearing sperm can be obtained. Fertilization in vitro seems to be possible with approximately that many normal sperm. We don't want to retrieve Mrs. Tilton's eggs and then not be able to fertilize them. Below 1 million, we have had very little success with fertilization. Mr. Tilton will have to return to Norfolk two more times at two-month intervals to give us a specimen."

"Mrs. Tilton," continued Dr. Garcia, "your ovaries now are not available to the laparoscope for egg retrieval. The right fallopian tube has covered the right ovary completely. The left ovary is held down by the left fallopian tube, which is attached by adhesions to the abdominal wall. We can remove these obstructions by a major surgical procedure called a laparotomy. An incision is made across the abdomen. We would remove your fallopian tubes and as many adhesions as possible. The ovaries would be moved over next to the uterus, and the uterus suspended so that the ovaries would be easily accessible by laparoscope for the retrieval of your eggs."

Garcia went on to explain that the surgery would require a week's stay in the hospital and a two-week recovery period. "That meant I couldn't have the surgery until my spring vacation the following March," says Nan. "I started planning it out . . . I'd have the operation in March, do the in vitro fertilization in July when school was out, and by April 1983 I could have a baby. In a year I could have a baby."

Before Nan and Todd left Norfolk, they made an appointment for Nan's laparotomy for March 9, 1982, provided Todd's sperm count was acceptable. The Tiltons went home to Sea Cliff with the same optimism they'd had when they went down to Norfolk. "But the pressure was really on me now," says Todd. "I had to keep my sperm count up there or they wouldn't take us."

Two more times Todd went down to Norfolk. On September 30, 1981, he made his second trip, and on November 17, he went down again. "It was a really easy trip," says Todd. "I'd leave work at the normal time, take the PATH train to Newark, catch People Express to Norfolk for twenty-nine dollars, have dinner, stay in the hotel overnight, get up early, ejaculate, drop off the container at Medical Tower, and catch the plane back. I'd be in my office by ten. The people in the office didn't even know, except I'm an open guy. I told them I was going down there for tests. Later they were in on the whole thing."

The first time Todd went down to provide a specimen he didn't call the in vitro clinic and reconfirm that he was coming. "That was a mistake," says Todd. "I rushed over to the office with the container of sperm, then had to stand around for twenty minutes waiting for a girl to come and get it. The stuff wasn't supposed to be more than thirty minutes old. And I didn't have that many sperm anyway, so I was paranoid. The next time I went down, I called the night before and had the girl there at the office waiting for me when I got there. That's what I mean about managing your own infertility situation. You have to take control of the situation and help the system work for you."

The laboratory analyses of Todd Tilton's sperm showed "4.7 million quick progressive sperm" on September 30, and 1.8 million on November 17. "This means," wrote Dr. Garcia on November 30, "Mr. Tilton oscillates between those values. We hope he will keep up at this level. Therefore, we could attempt in vitro fertilization to overcome your fertility . . . We can now think about doing the laparotomy on Mrs. Tilton, trying to fix her ovaries, and have her pelvis available for the first in vitro fertilization attempt in 1982."

The Tiltons had been accepted. "We were going to do it," says Nan. "We were right on schedule." She went to her calendars and wrote it all in.

Exactly one month later, Elizabeth Jordan Carr was born, the first baby conceived by in vitro fertilization at the Eastern Virginia Medical School in vitro clinic, the first born in the United States. She weighed five pounds, twelve ounces, and was pronounced "perfectly healthy" by her doctors at Norfolk General Hospital. The delivery was by Caesarian section, performed by Dr. Mason Andrews. The decision to perform a Caesarian was based on Dr. Andrews' concern about the small size of the baby, and because of the strain put on Mrs. Carr's body by her three previous ectopic pregnancies. Judy Carr's pregnancy had been monitored by her own obstetrician in Fitchburg, Massachusetts, and by Dr. Andrews, whom Mrs. Carr visited once a month in Norfolk.

Along with Dr. Andrews, Dr. Howard Jones, Jr., and his wife, Dr.

Georgeanna Jones, stood before the cameras of the national and international press, looking more like beaming grandparents than history-making professionals. "This morning," said Howard Jones, "at seven forty-six, a daughter was born to Mrs. Judith Carr, for whom it was impossible to become pregnant . . . except by the process of in vitro fertilization."

By the end of 1981, the Eastern Virginia Medical School VIP Program had achieved seven pregnancies, and one birth. In the second series of patients to be given the hormone stimulation, the pregnancy rate was 18 percent. The total number of babies conceived by in vitro fertilization born by December 1981 around the world was fifteen, the other fourteen having been born with Steptoe and Edwards in England and Carl Wood in Australia.

The prospects for in vitro fertilization at the end of 1981 were good. In the British medical journal *Lancet,* the editors suggested there was reason for optimism. The procedure, they said, may one day become simple and reliable enough to be handled on an outpatient basis. Judy and Roger Carr shared this vision of the future for in vitro fertilization. "By the time Elizabeth goes to school," said Judy Carr, "she won't be unique. There will be many children like her, conceived by in vitro fertilization."

The week before her spring vacation in March 1982, Nan Tilton spent every afternoon after school getting ready to go to Norfolk. She packed the Christening photograph, her scrapbook with the clippings, her photograph of Lesley Brown and baby Louise, and now a photograph of Judy and Roger Carr and baby Elizabeth. "They gave me hope, these women," says Nan. "I looked at them night and day and thought if it worked for them, it can work for me."

Nan and Todd left Sea Cliff on the morning of Monday, March 8. They went by car this time to Norfolk, to save money. Todd had taken a vacation from work to be with Nan. They arrived in Norfolk eight hours later with only minutes to spare before their two o'clock preoperative examination with Dr. Garcia. It was then that Nan discovered the laparotomy was a far more complicated and painful procedure than she had believed. "I thought it was going to be sort of like a Caesarian, a small incision and it would be over. But they were going to make an eight-inch incision across my stomach. This was major, major surgery."

"I will not lie to you," said Dr. Garcia, "your recovery will be very difficult."

Nan was admitted to Norfolk General Hospital that afternoon. Todd went to the hotel and checked in, then went back to the hospital to spend a few hours with Nan. Her surgery was scheduled for early the following morning. It was to be performed by two members of the Norfolk in vitro team, Dr. Anibal Acosta and Dr. Garcia.

Nan woke up from the operation the next day in terrible pain. "It really hurt," says Nan. "For eight days I lay in bed with this horrible pain. I couldn't eat, I couldn't sleep. I would be just going to sleep when a nurse would come in and wake me up to take my temperature." Nan finally got so upset at these intrusions that she wrote out a sign and put it on the door: "Keep Out! This Means You!" "I had to get some sleep or I'd go crazy." Todd tried to help her through it. "But whatever I suggested just made her mad," says Todd. "There was nothing I could do."

It was Dr. Garcia who helped Nan. Twice a day, early in the morning and at night, he came to see her.

"I don't know how he did it," says Nan. "He was always at the hospital. I've never seen such a dedicated man. He does all the in vitro surgeries, the sonograms, the laparoscopies, everything. He has to juggle so much information about so many women. But you feel that he's working only for you, to make in vitro happen for you. You just adore him."

The last day Nan was in the hospital, Dr. Garcia came into her room to give her a final checkup. The pain had subsided by then. Nan saw only what lay ahead. Tears came to her eyes. She grabbed Dr. Garcia's hand. "Thank you," she said, "for doing this, for giving us a chance." Dr. Garcia said, "Don't thank me now. You may have scarred over from the operation and we won't be able to get to your ovaries." Nan knew he was trying to prevent her from getting her hopes up. "He was always so careful not to be too encouraging," says Nan. "Only a very few women coming to Norfolk were getting pregnant. The odds were against us. It was his job to prepare his patients for disappointment." But Nan wasn't going to be discouraged or disappointed, she was going to get pregnant.

Nan and Todd drove home. Now there was nothing to do but wait, wait three months until the anesthesia was completely gone from her body, and Nan had healed from her operation. Then the attempt to conceive a baby, hers and Todd's baby, could begin.

After a two-week convalescence, Nan went back to Friends Academy, grateful for the hundredth time, and especially now, that she had something else to think about, someplace to express her ideas and channel her emotions. When the school year was over in the middle of June, Nan and

Todd joined a five-man crew on a friend's sailboat and raced in Block Island Race Week. They sailed by day and partied all night. Nan and Todd didn't know it, but it was to be their last vacation alone for a long time.

In Vitro
Fertilization Begins

Nan's menstruation began on the morning of Friday, July 2. Dr. Garcia had instructed the Tiltons to be at Medical Tower at 8:00 A.M. on the third day of Nan's period, even if it was a holiday or a weekend. This is Cycle Day 3. On a 28-day menstrual cycle, Day 3 is about 10 or 11 days before ovulation is expected to occur.

That Friday night Nan made dinner for their friends. They all stayed up late celebrating. Nan was too tired to clean up the kitchen. She and Todd piled the dishes in the sink and went to bed. They slept late the next morning, got up, cleaned the kitchen, and packed. They were very organized about it. "Our boating experience came in handy," says Todd. "We couldn't keep eating at the hotel with those prices, so we stocked up on provisions." They bought yogurt, soda, crackers and cheese, cereal, instant coffee—decaffeinated. Dr. Georgeanna Jones instructed the in vitro patients in the patient brochure that neither the husband nor wife should drink coffee, alcoholic beverages, nor should they smoke. "We know these things interfere with early embryonic development," says Dr. Georgeanna Jones, "so it's best to avoid them from the beginning."

The Tiltons packed the perishables in their boat cooler; they'd keep that in their room as a refrigerator. They also were taking an electric coffeepot, plastic plates and cups, utensils . . . "At least I'd know where to grab breakfast in the morning," says Nan.

Because extreme physical exercise was not permitted for in vitro patients, as fatigue could be detrimental to the process, there was going to be a lot of sitting around time. Nan and Todd each planned to take a project. Nan packed all the photographs she had taken for a slide presentation about Friends Academy that was to be her master's thesis in photography. She'd have plenty of time to edit the photographs while she was down there. Todd took some of his tax work.

Nan was going to have to be in Norfolk for three weeks. Todd was required to be there only on the day of the egg retrieval, and the day after, to provide the sperm. He had decided not to take vacation days from work. He was going to go down with Nan, get her settled in the hotel and stay with her for the first day or two, then fly back to New York for a few days, and come back for the egg retrieval. Nan's mother and Nan's brother had made plans to spend time with Nan in Norfolk after the embryo transfer.

There was no question this time that Nan and Todd would need their car. "We didn't want to have to depend on a taxi to get the semen to the hospital on time," says Nan, "or rely on a rented car that we didn't know. There was so much about the in vitro process that was uncertain, but there were some things we could do to make sure the conditions for its working were the best they could be. We'd gotten this far. We didn't want any slip-ups. Everything had to be as perfect as we could make it."

At four that afternoon, Nan and Todd loaded up the car and left for Norfolk. Nan drove the first four hours, Todd the second four hours. They arrived at the Omni Hotel at midnight. They piled their suitcases and supplies into a corner of their room and went to bed. At four o'clock in the morning, the lights went on suddenly and they awakened to find a man standing by their bed, looking as surprised to see them as they were to see him. A call to the front desk cleared up the situation. The clerk had given him the same hotel room by mistake. After that, Nan found it difficult to get back to sleep. At six-thirty she ordered breakfast brought to the room. By the time it came, she didn't have much of an appetite. While Todd was eating his breakfast, she looked over the information packet and schedule of procedures the clinic had sent her for about the twentieth time. She knew it all by heart, but somehow, being this close to beginning the in vitro treatment, it started to seem more real.

When the in vitro fertilization attempt begins, the VIP in vitro team takes over and manages the process of ovulation, starting with Cycle Day 3. Their goal is to be able to predict when ovulation will occur, not to the day, but to the hour, so that the eggs that are developing on the ovaries will be as mature as possible, and can be retrieved just prior to the moment when they would be ejected from the ovaries. The ovulation process is controlled daily by means of hormone injections that stimulate the eggs to mature. The progress of the developing follicles is monitored daily by blood tests, pelvic examination, and ultrasound examinations.

On Cycle Day 3, the in vitro patient is to report at eight o'clock to

Room 304 Medical Tower. There in the waiting room, the patient will find a box of test tubes with a label for the patient's name and the date. She is to fill this out and present it to the nurse, who will take a blood sample. The patient does this every morning. The blood test is one way the doctors have of judging the reaction of the ovaries to the hormone shots that will be administered on a daily basis. The blood is analyzed for the amount of estrogen. Estrogen is the hormone produced by the follicles of the ovary to prepare the cervix and uterus for fertilization. It is estrogen that triggers the release of the luteinizing hormone, which is responsible for ovulation.

By analyzing the patient's blood daily, the doctors can determine when ovulation is nearing. The level of estrogen rises as ovulation approaches, and it peaks about forty-eight hours before ovulation occurs. In a normal, unstimulated menstrual cycle, the estrogen level at its peak is 200 to 300 picograms per milliliter. In a hormone stimulated cycle, the estrogen level can reach 2,000 picograms per milliliter. The numbers are not significant except as an illustration of what a difference a hormone stimulated cycle makes. When more than one follicle is maturing on the ovaries, more estrogen is produced. An increase in the estrogen level in the blood is a sign that the hormone stimulation is working, and more than one follicle is developing on the ovaries.

After a blood sample is taken, the patient is given an injection in the upper buttock of pure FSH, follicle stimulating hormone, for the first two days of treatment. FSH is the hormone secreted by the pituitary gland. Its role in human reproduction is to stimulate the ovaries to produce an egg. The purpose of injecting in vitro patients with this hormone is to increase the amount of this hormone normally produced by the body in order to stimulate the ovaries to produce more than one egg.

In July 1982, when Nan and Todd Tilton began their in vitro attempt, patients were generally given only Pergonal, which is a combination of FSH and LH in a ratio of one to one, and which triggers ovulation. The change from a Pergonal-only drug protocol to a Pergonal-FSH protocol for the first two days of the hormone stimulation was made in early 1984. When Dr. Georgeanna Jones saw that some of the in vitro patients did not respond to the Pergonal stimulation, she substituted the morning injection of Pergonal with an injection of pure FSH for the first two days of the stimulation program. "At egg retrieval," she says, "we found we were retrieving many more eggs in these patients. Originally, with the Pergonal stimulation, we were retrieving an average of four eggs. An average of two and a half of these eggs were fertilizing and being transferred to the woman's uterus. By substituting an injection of pure FSH for those first two days, we were getting an average of six eggs at retrieval, and transferring an average of four and a half of them. The more eggs we retrieve, the more chance there is of their fertilizing, and the more embryos we can transfer into the uterus." What this means to the patient is that her chances of getting pregnant are increased.

On this first visit to Room 304 Medical Tower, the patient must sign consent forms for the various phases of the in vitro procedure. She must give the secretary her current address and telephone number so that doctors may reach her when necessary. Payment for the first phase of the in vitro process must be made then. This includes all the treatments administered until the day of egg retrieval. The total cost of this phase of the in vitro procedure in 1982 was $2,100. As of January 1985, the cost was $3,200. It is broken down into the following charges: Professional Charge, $2,000; Drugs, $300; Ultrasonography, $100; Endocrine Studies, $800.

In some cases, a semen specimen may be required of the husband on the first day. When all the treatments and payments have been completed on Cycle Day 3, the patient and her husband are invited to look at a videotape set up in the waiting room called "Introduction to the EVMS Vital Initiation of Pregnancy Program." The videotape is a recent addition to the VIP Program and did not exist when the Tiltons were there.

The videotape begins with an introduction by Dr. Howard Jones, Jr., and an explanation of the in vitro procedure. The tape includes a description of the procedures involved and actual videotape pictures from the operating room of an egg retrieval. Patients can see the ripe follicles on the ovaries being punctured and the eggs aspirated. This sequence is followed by a sequence on the laboratory procedures involved in preparing the egg and sperm for fertilization, and pictures of the fertilized embryos, in the two-cell stage, four-cell stage, and eight-cell stage. "It takes your breath away," said a recent patient, "to think that they can do that. It's like being offered a forbidden glimpse of the divine. I almost didn't want to look for fear of angering the gods and ruining my chances."

The first morning of treatment is now over. The patient is free now until four in the afternoon, when she must return for a second hormone injection. In the afternoon, she is given Pergonal.

The next day, Cycle Day 4, the procedure is exactly the same. Blood is drawn at 8:00 A.M. and the patient receives an injection of pure FSH in the morning and an injection of Pergonal in the afternoon. The blood sample is taken early in the morning so that there is time for it to be analyzed and the results examined before the four o'clock injection can be prescribed and administered.

Every afternoon at three, just before the afternoon injections, all the doctors and personnel on the in vitro team—Dr. Georgeanna Jones, who oversees the hormone stimulation protocol for each patient, Dr. Anibal Acosta, senior gynecologist, who works with couples who have subnormal sperm, Dr. Zev Rosenwaks, current director of the Institute, who specializes in reproductive medicine, Dr. Jairo Garcia, who evaluates the kinds of infertility problems that can be overcome by in vitro fertilization, and various fellows who stay with the VIP Program for a year to learn the in vitro technique, meet to evaluate each patient's situation. Dr. Howard Jones, Jr., does not participate in this conference. His role in the VIP Program is primarily administrative. He sees patients and helps out with laparoscopies and egg retrievals when the VIP caseload is heavy.

Depending on the levels of estrogen that are recorded in each patient's morning blood test, the doctors decide either to continue or to stop the FSH injection in the morning for that patient. If the estrogen level is rising, the FSH injections are stopped, but the patient continues to receive Pergonal injections in the afternoon.

On Cycle Day 6, when the menstrual period is over, blood is drawn, and then the patient is given her first pelvic examination and first ultrasound examination. The pelvic exam and ultrasound are two other methods by which the doctors can judge the effects of the hormone stimulation in a patient. In a pelvic examination, the doctors are concerned with two things: the status of the cervical mucus and the character of the cells of the vagina. Both undergo changes which signal the approach of ovulation. The cervical mucus becomes more abundant and transparent in appearance. The consistency of the mucus becomes stringy; it stretches into thin strands without breaking.

The cells of the vagina progress from an immature to mature state. The mature cells are recognizable because they are larger than the others and have a very distinct nuclei. When the ratio of mature to immature cells in the vagina reaches 30 percent, it is a sign that the patient is nearing ovulation.

These two factors, the cervical mucus and the cells of the vagina, constitute the *second* parameter after the blood test for determining when the patient's follicles are maturing. It is called the maturation index.

The third and last parameter in evaluating the effects of the hormone stimulation is the ultrasound examination. After three days of stimulation, follicles begin to grow on the surface of the ovaries. The developing follicles can actually be seen with the technique of ultrasound. Ultrasound is a technique which has been developed to look inside the human body. The way it works is as follows. Sound waves are reflected off body tissue and transmitted as a visual image on a television screen. Because sound waves travel best through body tissue and liquid rather than air, the patient is required to begin about two hours before her ultrasound exam to drink enough fluids to fill her bladder; six to eight eight-ounce glasses of water is about the right amount. She should have an empty bowel so that the view of her ovaries is not obstructed.

The ultrasound examination is conducted with the patient lying on her back. Mineral oil is rubbed over her abdomen to allow a cursor, a sort of flat pointer, to glide over the area and transmit the images of the internal abdominal cavity to the video screen. On the screen, the follicles appear as dark circles. By judging the size of the follicles, the doctors can get an idea of how close the patient is to ovulation. The conventional wisdom in in vitro technique is that the larger the follicle, the more mature is the egg it contains, and the more potential it has to fertilize and produce a pregnancy.

However, Dr. Georgeanna Jones feels strongly that ultrasound can be very misleading. "In our experience," she says, "large follicles can produce bad oocytes [eggs] and small follicles can produce good ones. If we didn't take the small follicles during our egg retrievals, we'd miss a third of our pregnancies." In addition, the number of follicles seen during an ultrasound exam very often proves at egg retrieval not to have been accurate. "There might be something in the way, obscuring our view of the ovaries by ultrasound," explains Dr. Georgeanna Jones. "Ultrasound gives us only a rough indication of the number of eggs we should expect to find."

For the next three to eight days of an in vitro patient's treatment, all three of these parameters are evaluated every day—blood, pelvic exam, and ultrasound. When the estrogen level appears to be peaking, when the cells of the vagina and the cervical mucus have "shifted" to preovulatory status, and when the ultrasound shows that follicles are good-sized—fourteen to fifteen millimeters in diameter—then the patient is judged to be ready for her egg retrieval. "You can't look at any one of those parameters alone," emphasizes Dr. Georgeanna Jones. "You have to look at all three of them. Ultrasound is the least reliable. If I had to do without one of those parameters, it would be ultrasound."

This is one significant way in which the Norfolk VIP Program differs from many other clinics currently practicing in vitro fertilization in the United States. Many of the other in vitro programs rely almost exclusively on ultrasound to judge a patient's readiness for egg retrieval. "I don't know why they can't do a pelvic exam," says Dr. Georgeanna Jones. "It's so simple. It's the only one of the parameters that doesn't require any fancy technology. I think the shift of the maturation index is the most important thing to go by."

"We used to do pelvic exams," says a representative of a university in vitro program in New England, "but it took too long." Dr. Georgeanna Jones feels that this may be one reason why other clinics are not as successful in achieving pregnancies as they are at Norfolk.

The Joneses have had enough experience now to be able to see certain patterns in the response of their patients to the hormone stimulation, and they are able to gauge their chances of success on the basis of these patterns. "The pattern of response that has the best pregnancy rate," explains Dr. Georgeanna Jones, "is one in which the estrogen level rises continually over the period in which the hormones are being administered. This pattern we call the A Pattern.

"If we see that the patient's estrogen level plateaus or drops down during the hormone stimulation, it usually means that the follicles are degenerating, and the chances of retrieving a good egg are not as good. This pattern of response we call the G Pattern. A third pattern, the B Pattern, shows the patient's estrogen level rising, but then when the Pergonal is stopped and the HCG injection is given, the estrogen level goes down, then up again. This means we will have immature follicles at the egg retrieval. We prefer the Pattern A response; we have a better chance of getting mature eggs. But we will take Patterns G and B to laparoscopy too."

In some cases, after the first several days of the hormone stimulation, it becomes clear that the patient is not responding appropriately, or there are complications. It has become the practice at Norfolk to cancel these patients before they reach the egg retrieval phase. One reason for cancellation is an inappropriate response to hormone stimulation. The estrogen level may go up too early, or it goes down to half of what it was the previous day and stays low. Cysts may also be found on a patient's ovaries, or follicles may be developing on an inaccessible part of a patient's ovaries. These patients too are canceled. All canceled patients are rescheduled for another in vitro attempt. In the interim, the in vitro team works out another approach to the patient's hormone stimulation protocol, either changing the dosage or the type of medication given.

"In the beginning," says Dr. Garcia, "we were proud to be treating everybody, without cancellations. I think, knowing what we do now, it is foolish not to cancel someone when her chances of getting pregnant are not as high as they could be. Of course, patients are very upset when they are sent home. But when they come back for the next attempt, and respond to the new stimulation protocol we give them, they are grateful because they understand they have a much better chance of getting pregnant."

When all three parameters indicate that the patient is nearing ovulation, the Pergonal injections are stopped. "We have now accomplished our goal," says Dr. Garcia, "the recruitment of eggs and follicular development. Then we wait." The patient is still required to come to the office at Medical Tower every morning for a blood test. Fifty hours after the Pergonal has been stopped, the patient is given an injection of the hormone HCG, human chorionic gonadotropin. HCG is similar to luteinizing hormone; its purpose is to mimic the body's normal surge of LH in midcycle, which causes the mature egg to burst from the ovary.

Thirty-six hours after the HCG injection, the eggs are mature and ready to be retrieved. At that time, the laparoscopy is performed, and the eggs are removed from the ovaries and taken to the laboratory. At Norfolk, the egg retrieval is done most often on Cycle Day 11. The timing of the HCG injection and the laparoscopy is one of the most crucial factors in the success of the in vitro procedure. If the eggs are harvested too soon, they may not be ready to fertilize. If it is done too late, ovulation may have already occurred and the eggs vanished into the abdominal cavity.

The goal then of this first phase of the in vitro procedure is to stimulate the ovaries to produce more than one egg, and then to determine when the eggs are mature in order to be able to retrieve them at the right time. While the procedure explained above is the general procedure for egg recruitment at the Eastern Virginia Medical School's VIP Program, every patient is treated individually. The response of each patient to the hormone stimulation is quite different. "Therefore," reads the patient brochure, "do not expect equal results in regard to time, duration of treatment, number and quality of eggs that are retrieved. Each case is different. Remember: The book about you has not yet been written."

Prior to July 1982, the Norfolk clinic had treated a total of 142 patients in four six-week sessions. That is about thirty-five patients per session. Each cycle of in vitro patients is made up of roughly half new patients and half repeaters, patients who have not gotten pregnant in previous attempts. There is no limit to the number of times a patient may return for the in vitro procedure. Some have come back seven times before they have gotten pregnant. The overall pregnancy rate at the EVMS

VIP Program at that time was 13 percent, but the pregnancy rate for the clinic's previous cycle of patients was 15 percent. "We learned more and more with each series of patients," says Dr. Howard Jones, Jr. When Nan and Todd Tilton came to Norfolk, the clinic was treating its fifth series of patients.

Nan and Todd Tilton arrived at Medical Tower a few minutes before eight that first morning. It was a Sunday, the Fourth of July. There wasn't a soul on the streets of downtown Norfolk at that hour. Nan and Todd got off the elevator on the third floor and went right to Room 304. Nan opened the door and to her astonishment, she saw that the room was full of people. People were sitting on the floor, standing against the wall; she and Todd could hardly get into the room. "Here I was, anticipating a private celebration with Dr. Garcia," says Nan, "and there were all these people. It was a bit frightening."

Nan Tilton was the nineteenth patient to enter the VIP Program in Series V. There would be forty-six patients in Series V who would begin treatment between June 29 and August 2. Any patient accepted for Series V who did not reach Cycle Day 3 within this time period would have to wait for Series VI, which would begin in September.

Because it was July 4, there was no receptionist in the waiting room to tell the Tiltons what to do. One of the women patients noticed the Tiltons' confusion. "You're new, aren't you," she said, smiling. She showed Nan the box of test tubes for the blood test and told her how to fill out the label. "Everyone in the room was looking at us," says Nan. "We felt very conspicuous." Nan and Todd took up a position near the door and tried to look casual, and after a few minutes the other patients lost interest in them. That was when Nan started sneaking looks at the other couples. "I'd only known one other person who had an infertility problem," says Nan, "and here was a whole roomful of them."

As Nan looked around the room, she saw a variety of expressions. She saw hope in some faces, fear and anxiety in others. She saw determination, and she saw resignation. She decided right then that she would never reach the point of resignation. She was going to make in vitro fertilization work for her and Todd if she had to work at it twenty-four hours a day.

About ten minutes later, a doctor unfamiliar to the Tiltons came to the door of the waiting room. "Who's first today?" One by one, the women went in for their shots and blood tests and left. The women who had come with their husbands left with other couples; the other women seemed to leave in pairs or threesomes. The waiting room cleared out very rapidly. Nan and Todd waited until the end to go in. While they were waiting, they struck up a conversation with a couple standing next to them, Andrea and Bob Nelson. "I could tell they were New Yorkers," says Todd. It turned out they were from Roslyn, Long Island. This was their second day in Norfolk. Andrea Nelson was on Cycle Day 4.

After the Nelsons were finished, the Tiltons went in. Nan handed the nurse her blood tube. The nurse looked at a list hanging on the wall and found Nan's name. "I was relieved to see it was there," says Nan. The nurse took Nan's blood, then sent the Tiltons down the short hallway to Dr. Themis Mantzauinos, known as Dr. T., a VIP fellow, for Nan's injection. "I need your right buttock," he said. "Pull up your skirt and pull down your pants." Nan was given an injection of Pergonal. The clinic had not yet begun to use pure FSH in their routine stimulation protocol. "You're done," said Dr. T. "Is that all?" asked Nan. "Where's Dr. Garcia?" asked Todd. "He's doing laparoscopies today; he'll be in tomorrow," said the doctor and the Tiltons left.

On the way back to the hotel in the car, Nan began to feel strange. "I felt sort of high, light-headed," she says. "I couldn't believe I was having a reaction from the shot so soon." Nan and Todd went right up to their room. Nan made sandwiches out of the food they'd brought with them and they watched tennis matches on TV until Nan fell asleep.

A few hours later, Nan got up, changed her clothes, put on fresh makeup, and at four she and Todd went back over to Medical Tower for her second injection of Pergonal. While they were waiting, they made a date with the Nelsons to meet back at the Omni Hotel afterward for drinks at the bar. The Nelsons were staying at the Omni too. Since alcoholic beverages were forbidden for all of them, they ordered soft drinks and onion rings, which were to become staples in the women's diets for the next several weeks. Afterward, Nan and Todd went back up to their room and Nan slept again. "Those first few days it seems I was always sleeping," says Nan. "The injections made me sleepy. After a while I got used to them I guess; they didn't bother me as much."

That night Nan and Todd drove thirty miles to Virginia Beach for dinner and Fourth of July fireworks. "You can imagine what Fourth of July was like in a military town," says Todd. "Every marine and sailor stationed in the vicinity of Norfolk was there." "And every one of them was with his family," says Nan. "Mothers, fathers, little girls and little boys, all tan and healthy, dressed in their summer shorts and sun dresses."

Then Nan saw the picture that would remain with her for the duration of her stay in Norfolk. "I'm a photographer. I see everything in still images." It was a little boy sitting on his father's shoulders. "He was the perfect copy of his father," says Nan. "They were both wearing baseball hats and baseball shirts. My heart jumped. That was why Todd and I were in Norfolk. We were going to have a little boy and he was going to be the image of Todd."

On the drive back to Norfolk, Nan and Todd talked over their first day in the VIP Program and they decided that they were going to ask to see Dr. Garcia the next day. "We were feeling a little left out in the cold," says Todd. "By this time we were used to dealing with our infertility problem aggressively. We wanted to make sure the VIP doctors knew we were there, that we were part of the special program for husbands with low sperm counts, and we wanted them to know we weren't going to get lost in the shuffle."

The next morning, Monday, July 5, Nan and Todd got to the office a little early for Nan's blood test and injection. The receptionist was in. They asked to see Dr. Garcia and she took them right into his office. "As soon as we saw him," says Nan, "everything was fine. We knew he wasn't going to forget us or get us mixed up with someone else." Dr. Garcia told Todd that he would have to be available to provide another semen sample on Wednesday morning at eight. "We must be sure your count is still over one million," said Dr. Garcia. "You must give us the specimen now so that there will be enough time to produce sperm again before you must provide the specimen to fertilize Mrs. Tilton's eggs." This meant that Todd had to stay two days longer than he had planned. He called his office to tell them he wouldn't be in until Wednesday afternoon.

After Nan's blood test and Pergonal injection, she and Todd went back to the hotel. Nan didn't feel quite as sleepy as she had the day before, so they decided to go down to the pool. The swimming pool at the Omni was like any hotel swimming pool. It was small, meant for transient guests. But the women VIP patients had turned it into the focal point of all their experiences, past and present, in trying to achieve pregnancy.

The in vitro couples identified each other immediately; they had already seen each other in the waiting room at Medical Tower. Nan was hesitant to run right over to the group that had already drawn their lounge chairs together, but Todd went over and introduced himself. The other couples moved their chairs to make room for Nan and Todd. "Is this your first time?" was always the first question put to a newly arrived couple. Nan heard stories that morning at the swimming pool that made her hair stand on end. "Some women had already been there four times and they still hadn't gotten pregnant," says Nan. "There were some women who had had three embryos transferred and it didn't work."

Todd was surprised at how easily the men and women, perfect strangers, talked about such intimate things with each other. "These were things we'd never talked about to a living soul, except each other," says Todd, "and here we were talking about them with strangers and laughing about it." Throughout Nan and Todd's stay in Norfolk, however, they never told anyone that Todd had an infertility problem. "We let Todd be the big macho guy," says Nan, "like everyone else. He was going to fertilize my eggs." None of the men with low sperm counts talked about it. "You usually knew who they were, though," says Todd, "because their wives eventually told the other women, and the women told their husbands." "But no one ever talked about it in public," says Nan. "The wives were very protective of the husbands with low sperm counts."

For Nan, the talking was a heady experience. She was absolutely exhilarated to be able to share her experience with someone else. "I'd been the only one for so long . . . and here were fifteen women all in one place."

"It's like coming home," said one in vitro patient recently who had returned to Norfolk for her third try at in vitro fertilization. "I feel as though I belong to a sisterhood when I'm here. It's the only place I don't feel weird."

Some couples come from as far away as South America to try in vitro fertilization at the Norfolk program. There are couples from Egypt, the Philippines, Europe; some didn't speak any English at all, but there is an immediate bond among in vitro patients generated by the fact that they have in common the most important thing in their lives, their inability to bear children.

At the pool that day, Nan and Todd found out that the doctors had stopped Andrea Nelson's Pergonal injections that morning. It meant that Andrea would get her HCG shot the next day, and go for her egg retrieval laparoscopy on Thursday. "It gave me goose bumps to think Andrea was that close," says Nan.

But instead of being optimistic about the prospect of her egg retrieval, Andrea Nelson was a nervous wreck. This was her second attempt at in vitro fertilization. She'd been among the Joneses' first series of patients in 1980, when they were still using the natural cycle. She was their eleventh patient. She'd had an ectopic pregnancy in one fallopian tube and the tube was removed. The other tube was blocked and one ovary was obscured. At that time Norfolk had not achieved a single pregnancy.

Before she was accepted by the VIP Program, she had to have the other tube removed. She had had to remain in the hospital for the entire three weeks of her in vitro treatment; the doctors monitored the development of her egg by taking blood every hour. She never got as far as the transfer. The egg that the in vitro team retrieved during her laparoscopy did not fertilize. It had taken her two years to get up the courage to come back to Norfolk and try again. She just could not bear the disappointment if it should fail this time too.

At about three o'clock, the in vitro patients at the pool gradually drifted up to their rooms to get ready to go over to the office for their four o'clock injections. The experienced couples knew just how long it took, to the minute, to go upstairs, change, and get to the office. They tended to dawdle longer at the pool. Every one of the women came down to the lobby fifteen minutes later in different clothes and fresh makeup. "It was a real fashion show," says Todd. "Every day the gals showed up in a different outfit. Some of the women came down there with trunks of clothes."

"There's nothing else to do," said a recent in vitro patient. "You have time to do your nails and put on makeup, go to the hairdresser." "Clothes are an outlet for many of the women's frustrations," says Nan. "You don't have kids, you buy clothes."

By three forty-five most of the couples had left the hotel. Those who didn't have cars always found someone to take them over to the office. At four-thirty Nan had her second Pergonal injection that day. "I felt my ovaries twinge after that one," says Nan. She felt sleepy afterward and took a rest before dinner. Nan and Todd drove to Virginia Beach again that night for dinner, and the Nelsons went with them.

"We really had a lovely evening," says Nan. "Todd and I liked them. But there was something about Andrea's attitude toward the in vitro process that bothered me. She was working herself into a state of real fear. She was calling her mother every day. Andrea was afraid of the surgery, afraid of the anesthetic . . . I thought if she didn't change her attitude fast, in vitro was not going to work for her."

Andrea Nelson's psychological problem was exacerbated by the fact that the hormone stimulation had worked very quickly on her. She had been receiving the Pergonal only three days before the doctors stopped the injections, and made plans for her egg retrieval. In most patients, the egg retrieval came around Cycle Day 11. Andrea Nelson was going to have her laparoscopy on Cycle Day 9.

The next morning, Cycle Day 5, Nan went to the office alone for her blood test and injection. After two days of hormone stimulation, her blood test showed that her estrogen level on the second day was slightly higher than the day before. Nan went back to the hotel and found that Todd had gone down to the swimming pool. "Todd was going crazy, just sitting around," says Nan. Nan did some hand laundry in the room, then went down to the pool to join Todd.

At the pool that day, Nan met Shari Johnson. Nan had seen her at the office. Shari had known since she was seventeen that she was infertile. She'd had emergency surgery when she was a teenager and her fallopian tubes had been blocked ever since. She got married knowing that the only way she would be able to have a baby was by in vitro fertilization. "As soon as Lesley Brown had her baby," said Shari, "I knew that was what I was going to do." She too carried a picture of Lesley Brown and baby Louise as inspiration. Nan felt she had found a soulmate. Here was someone as determined as she was. "We encouraged each other," says Nan.

That afternoon, Nan drove Shari over to the office for their shots. It made her just as sleepy as it did the day before. "I had to have my usual afternoon nap," says Nan. They had dinner again with the Nelsons and went to see *E.T.* Afterward they went back to the hotel for dessert and decaffeinated coffee at the piano bar in the lobby. The chairs were deep and comfortable, the music soothing; outside the lights of the harbor twinkled, and Nan felt a sense of well-being.

Two weeks later, during the long stretch of uncertainty after the embryo transfer, when the husbands had all gone home, this piano bar was to be the women's refuge, a place to escape from the tension of waiting to know if they were pregnant or not. It was the time when all the enjoyment that could be gotten from leisurely dinners at elegant restaurants had been exhausted, all the stories exchanged and reassuring words used up, and there remained only the four impersonal walls of a hotel room and a television babbling nonstop to drown out the anxiety. It was the time when every woman's worst moments of her infertility experience came back to haunt her. So the women gathered there in the bar, speaking little, taking comfort from each other's presence.

As Nan looked around her that night, she saw those women . . . waiting. She could read in their faces what awaited her, the hope tempered by fear as each hurdle of the in vitro process was met and overcome, then the waiting and fear mounting again until the time came to meet the next hurdle. Nan shivered involuntarily, reaching out for Todd's hand. She would not be afraid. It was going to work for them, she believed it. . . .

The next day, Wednesday, July 7, Nan was on Cycle Day 6. Todd had to deliver his semen specimen to the hospital that morning by eight.

He took the car and Nan drove over to Medical Tower with the Nelsons. According to the schedule Nan had been given on her first day in Norfolk, this was the day she was going to have her first pelvic examination and her first ultrasound.

After she had had her blood drawn and the nurse had given her the Pergonal injection, Nan went into the examining room. Dr. T. did the exam. Nan took off her pants and lay down on the examining table on her back. Dr. T. inserted a speculum to keep the vagina open and took a sample of her cervical mucus and a sample of the tissue from the walls of her vagina. He could tell right away that Nan's cervical mucus was becoming more abundant. "You have mucus," he said. "That's very good." Nan felt as if she'd gotten an A+ on a school exam. "I was doing all right," says Nan gleefully.

Now Nan had to drink six glasses of water for her ultrasound exam. She'd already started at breakfast, but the doctors told her it wasn't enough, she had to drink more. Most of the women were gone by the time she was ready. It was Dr. Garcia who gave her the ultrasound exam. Nan's tension melted instantly when she saw him. "Hello, Dr. Garcia," she said, looking for the spark of sympathy in his eyes that connected him so intimately to each of his patients. "What happens next?" Nan asked.

Quietly, Dr. Garcia showed her how the ultrasound worked. Nan lay down on the examining table on her back and pulled down her pants to below her abdomen. Dr. Garcia squirted the mineral oil onto her stomach; it was cold. Nan gasped in surprise. "Excuse me," apologized Dr. Garcia. "We usually warm the oil first." He moved the ultrasound cursor over her abdomen and suddenly, on the television screen next to the table, Nan saw two vaguely round areas with little dark craters in them. "It looked like a photograph of the moon," says Nan.

Dr. Garcia explained that the round areas were her ovaries, and each of the dark spots was a follicle developing. A little arrow suddenly flew across the screen. "The arrow measures the size of the follicles," said Dr. Garcia. As the arrow traced the width of each follicle, numbers flashed onto the screen. "See," pointed out Dr. Garcia, "there are follicles developing on both ovaries. That is very good." Nan left Medical Tower that morning with her spirits soaring. "Everything was happening just right," says Nan.

Nan met Todd back at the hotel with her good news. Todd was leaving that afternoon to go back to New York, so they went to the supermarket to stock up on provisions for Nan, then Nan drove Todd to the airport. It was going to feel strange not to have him there with her, but at the same time Nan was looking forward to being with the girls. Nan worried the whole way out to the airport that she wouldn't get back to Medical Tower in time for her four o'clock injection. "I was afraid something would go wrong," says Nan. She did get back, though, in time.

The three nurses who draw the patients' blood and give the injections every day are the members of the Norfolk in vitro team who see the patients most often. While the doctors rotate daily, depending on who is in the operating room doing laparoscopies and transfers, the nurses, Jan Coleridge, Linda Ellis, and Doris, remain at Medical Tower.

"We see the patients thirty to forty times while they're here," said Jan Coleridge, clinic nurse coordinator. She was with the Norfolk clinic for two years. She has since left the program. The nurse's role, however, is more than just giving shots to the patients every day. She is the person the women come to when they have questions, when they have fears, when they're upset. "Our program doesn't have a psychologist on staff," said Jan. "We fulfill that need."

"When we're drawing their blood, that's when they tell us their problems," says Doris, who has been with the VIP Program since its inception. "They say they've heard that someone has been canceled, or someone else is going for her egg retrieval on Day 9 and they're already on Day 9, and they haven't even stopped their injections yet. Usually we can help them just by listening and repeating over and over again that every patient is different. By the time they get here, our patients have already been through so much. They don't need people fussing at them. They need tender, loving care."

The nurses also recognize that every series of patients that comes through the VIP Program has its own personality. "Some groups are quiet, they're very compliant, no questions," said Jan. "Other cycles, we have real go-getters, very aggressive patients who want to know everything you're doing and why. One group I remember, there were two ladies with a strong personality conflict. It rubbed off on all the other patients, and they ended up taking sides."

So far, Nan had not had occasion to avail herself of the nurses' counsel. "My method," says Nan, "was to stay cool, and not get upset about anything ahead of time. I hated having my blood drawn, but I wasn't going to get upset about it until I went in there. *Then* I got nervous, but soon it was over. I didn't think about it again until the next time. So many women let their anxiety build up from one treatment to the next, just accumulating it until they had to let it out. That made all the other women nervous. I didn't pay any attention to anyone else. One day a woman fainted while Jan was taking her blood. There was a crash. We heard it out in the waiting room. Andrea Nelson freaked out. I told her, 'Forget it. Don't think about it. It doesn't have anything to do with you.' "

That night after Todd left, Nan went out to dinner with Andrea and Bob Nelson. Andrea had to be at the hospital at eleven that night for her HCG shot. After dinner the Nelsons dropped Nan off at the hotel, and she went up to her room. "It was the first time I was going back to my room without Todd," says Nan. "I really missed him. I didn't like having to stay in my room all by myself."

When Nan got to her door, there was a loud party going on in the rooms at the end of the corridor. "The Navy had moved in," says Nan. "There were so many guys, they were partying in the hall." As soon as they saw Nan, they asked her to join them. "They're propositioning me while I'm unlocking the door," says Nan. "And I could smell pot everywhere. I didn't smoke pot and I didn't want to smell pot; I didn't want any of that pot getting into my body; that was the last thing I wanted while I was trying to get pregnant."

Nan turned around and went right back downstairs to the night manager and asked to have her room changed immediately. "I was screaming at the guy on the other side of the desk," says Nan, "demanding a room. He probably thought the in vitro women were nuts. I think we were, with all those hormones we were getting." The manager never considered not responding to her request. He found a room for Nan on another floor. He told her to get her things together, he'd send a porter up to help her move them.

Nan went back up to her room and looked around at all the food and clothes and papers and things spread all over . . . "Every drawer was stuffed, I'd been living there for four days already, it was home. I was all alone. I couldn't imagine how I was going to move everything . . ." Nan took a deep breath, gathered herself together, and went back down to the lobby. She told the night manager she needed *two* rooms that night, one for her and one for her things. She would move everything to the new room the next day. " 'I can't possibly do that,' he said. 'You have to,' I said. 'My husband's not here, I've been shot up with hormones . . .' and then I started crying. The manager said, 'Okay, okay, Mrs. Tilton, we'll take care of it. Just take what you need up to the other room, lock the door, and you can move the rest tomorrow, but before 11 A.M.' "

By the time Nan got back to her room, the party had broken up and Nan decided to sleep in her old room. She changed rooms the next morning, but she didn't feel comfortable about it. "I was very superstitious," says Nan. "I thought it might affect the success of the in vitro treatment. I'd been happy in that room. I didn't want to change anything."

The next morning was Nan's Cycle Day 8. She had been in Norfolk now for five days. "It seemed like eons," says Nan. She and Andrea went over to the office together for their blood tests. Even though Andrea had had her Pergonal stopped, she still had to go to the office in the morning for blood tests. The in vitro team had to know if the follicles were responding to the HCG injection, and that they would be ready for retrieval on Friday.

The waiting room at Medical Tower that morning was buzzing. "Did you hear?" said Shari as soon as Nan and Andrea walked in the door. "Maria is pregnant." "Oh my God," squealed Nan, "it's real. This thing works." Nan was getting impatient now for her laparoscopy to come.

Her turn came that morning. "We're stopping your Pergonal today," said Doris. "Come back this afternoon for an ultrasound exam." "I was so excited," says Nan. Then Dr. Garcia motioned her into the examining room. "What's happening?" asked Nan. "Am I ready for my egg retrieval?" Dr. Garcia smiled. "We have to give you a pelvic exam," he said. "Lie down." Dr. Garcia took mucus and vaginal samples. "We're getting close," he said. "We'll know for sure this afternoon after we get the results of this morning's blood test." Nan waited for Andrea and Shari, and they went out to breakfast to celebrate their progress.

That afternoon Nan went back to the office with Shari. Shari had been having headaches after her injections. When she went in to get her shot, she told Jan. Jan wasn't surprised. "Other patients have complained of headaches too, and even vomiting. Don't worry. Take some Tylenol if it gets really bad, and fill out this questionnaire. The manufacturer asked us to give them to our patients so that they can find out how prevalent these side effects are."

While Shari was with Jan, Nan was waiting for her ultrasound exam. Dr. Garcia was doing the ultrasounds too that day. When Nan's turn came, she lay down right away on the table, then looked up expectantly. She felt her heart leap with fear. "I could tell right away there was something bothering him," says Nan. "Is something wrong?" she asked. Dr. Garcia did not answer right away. He squirted the mineral oil on her abdomen in silence and almost absentmindedly moved the cursor over her stomach, watching the video screen. "I just had to tell a couple that we could not continue with our in vitro attempt," said Dr. Garcia gravely. "She had already ovulated."

Nan let out her breath slowly and felt herself trembling with relief. "I thought something was wrong with me," said Nan. Dr. Garcia turned off the ultrasound and turned to Nan. "We're definitely stopping your Pergonal. You will get your HCG shot tomorrow; we will probably do your laparoscopy on Sunday." "Really?" squealed Nan. "It's really going to happen?" Dr. Garcia allowed himself a little smile. "We will continue to monitor your situation," he said. "If it continues to progress, then we will do the laparoscopy."

Nan left the examining room and rushed out to tell Shari, who was waiting for her. "I'm having my laparoscopy Sunday," said Nan. Shari hugged her. She was happy for Nan, but she was anxious. Her injections still hadn't been stopped yet. "Don't worry," Nan said. "Remember what Dr. Garcia says. Don't listen to what any other women tell you. Listen to him. He'll keep you up to date on your case." Shari smiled gratefully.

Nan went right back to the hotel to call Todd. He was required to be in Norfolk the day of the laparoscopy to provide the sperm to fertilize the eggs that were retrieved. He would take the Friday night flight from Newark and arrive at seven-thirty. He was going to stay with Nan until after the embryo transfer. After that, Nan's mother was coming down to Norfolk to stay with her.

Nan and Shari and another in vitro patient named Rebecca went out to dinner that night on Military Highway, where there were a lot of fast food places and steak houses. "We all felt guilty about spending so much money on dinners," says Nan. "We decided to go cheap that night." When the women got together, they never talked about anything but in vitro—who had gone for surgery, how many eggs did she have, how many were transferred, who was sent home, who was getting FSH, who wasn't, whose husbands were staying. "All we were concerned about for ourselves," says Nan, "was, would they get eggs from us? Were they going to get two eggs? That was what everyone was hoping for, two good eggs. With two eggs, you had twice as much of a chance of getting pregnant."

The more the women talked that night, the more they preyed on each other's fears. "The fact is," said Rebecca, "only one of us at this table will get pregnant. Those are the odds." Shari immediately burst into tears. "Looking back," says Nan, "I can see why it happened. We were all on the verge of hysteria; our hormones were going wild. There was the tension of waiting, and not knowing what was happening. Here we were sitting around doing nothing because that's what we were supposed to be doing, while the doctors manipulated our bodies to make them pregnant. Everything was riding on that. Rebecca made us confront the fact that the odds were against us. Only one in three of us was going to get pregnant. But it was wrong of her to remind us. I could take it, but Shari couldn't."

The next morning when Nan and Shari went over to the office for their blood tests, Shari found out she was going for her laparoscopy on Sunday too. Shari was greatly relieved. Now she too could be excited. She went back to the hotel to call her husband. Nan saw the whole day stretching before her with nothing to do. Todd wouldn't be arriving until that evening. She felt a little panicky. She needed something to distract her. Her slide presentation was the last thing she wanted to think about. The box of slides she'd brought down to work on was still packed away. She hadn't opened it once since she'd been down in Norfolk. "I couldn't do anything that required any concentration," says Nan. "I'd turned into a real flake."

Nan took the car and drove over to a shopping mall on the outskirts of Norfolk. She wandered around the stores for a while, then found a handwork store. "I was thinking, What am I going to do all those days after the surgery and the transfer when I'm waiting around to find out if I'm pregnant? I wanted something to do with my hands." She bought a Quick Stitch stitchery kit to make a pillow. "I was getting ready," says Nan, "to sit on my nest."

The heat outside was unbearable. Nan went back to the hotel and got into bed with her stitchery kit and some snacks. At two forty-five she went over to Medical Tower for her ultrasound with Dr. Garcia. "Very good," he said, looking at the screen. Nan began to feel butterflies in her stomach. It was so close now. Dr. Garcia gave Nan a prescription for the HCG injection. He instructed her to take the prescription to the pharmacy at Norfolk General Hospital and get it filled before five. The injection would be administered by a nurse at Norfolk General Hospital at eleven that night. The HCG had to be kept refrigerated until then. Then Dr. Garcia sent Nan to Linda Lynch to fill out hospital admission forms and a consent form that gives the doctors permission to perform the laparoscopy. This is routine practice with any surgical procedure. Linda also gave Nan a diagram of Norfolk General Hospital, with the admitting area, pharmacy, and nurses station, where she was to get her injection, all clearly marked.

Nan and Shari went over to the pharmacy together afterward to get their prescriptions filled. The pharmacist would refrigerate the HCG for them until that night. Then they went back to the hotel to visit Andrea Nelson, who had had her laparoscopy the day before. They had gotten two eggs. "She was very lucky," says Nan. To Nan's surprise, Andrea wasn't at the hotel. Bob told them that Andrea had gotten very sick from the anesthesia and the doctors wanted her to remain in the hospital overnight. "It worried me," says Nan. "She shouldn't have had that bad a reaction. It made me think she was working against herself somehow. She should have been out of that hospital in four hours and back in her room resting so that when her embryos were put inside her, they would stay."

It was time then for Nan to go to the airport to get Todd. "I was so glad to see him," says Nan. "It put everything into perspective. Being with the girls was all right, but with Todd there I could really focus on what was important—*me* getting pregnant." Nan and Todd had dinner alone in their room that night, then at ten-thirty they met Shari and her husband in the lobby and went over to the hospital together for the HCG shots. "I was worried about this shot," says Nan. "All the girls said it was very painful. They use a needle about a foot long and stick it in your rear end, which by this time is full of pinpricks . . ."

The hospital was silent at that hour of the night. The four of them went first to the pharmacy to get their medicine, then up to the fourth-floor nurses station in A Wing where the injections were to be administered. "A Wing was the maternity section," says Nan. "It was almost too much to bear. We had to walk past the nursery to get there . . . all those babies, someone else's babies."

Nan and Shari had to wait in the birthing room to get their shots. "It was the room in which the women having natural childbirth delivered their babies," explains Nan. "It didn't look like a hospital room. There was a big easy chair for Daddy; and a mural on one wall of mountains for the woman to look at while she's in labor, and a picture of a baby on the ceiling." The VIP Program has now moved its operating room and laboratory to the first floor in order to spare its patients this emotional ordeal.

At eleven o'clock on the dot, the nurse came in to give Nan her injection. It hurt, but not as much as Nan expected. The Tiltons waited until Shari got her shot at eleven-thirty, then they all went back to the hotel.

On Saturday, July 10, Cycle Day 9, one day before her egg retrieval, Nan woke up and took her temperature as she had done every day since she had been down in Norfolk, and was horrified to see that her temperature had shot up. This was the result of the HCG injection she'd been given the night before, but Nan didn't know that. "I was petrified," says Nan. "I thought it meant I'd already ovulated." She wanted to see Dr. Garcia immediately, but before she could go over to Medical Tower, she and Shari were required to be at the hospital for preoperative checkups. "The nurse took blood and urine samples," says Nan, "and told us to be at the hospital at six-thirty on Sunday morning." They were then directed to the administrative offices, where they paid a one-thousand-dollar deposit for hospital expenses.

Nan didn't say anything to Shari about her fears, but the more she committed herself to the laparoscopy, the more frightened she became. "I kept thinking I was doing this paperwork for nothing. I was sure Dr. Garcia was going to send me home."

When Shari and Nan finished at the hospital, they went over to Medical Tower for their pelvic exams and ultrasounds. The office was so crowded that Linda Lynch told them to come back later. Nan was going crazy now. "I wanted to know," says Nan, "but I also didn't want to know." She and Shari went to the coffee shop across from Medical Tower to pass the time. Nan could not swallow a thing.

An hour later, they went back to the office and Dr. Garcia was ready for them. "Who's first?" he asked. "Me," said Nan before Shari had a chance. Nan decided she would not tell him about her fears. If they were unfounded, she'd be embarrassed. Also she did not want to present even the slightest hint of negativity to Dr. Garcia. "I felt it might jinx the whole thing," she says.

In the examining room, Dr. Garcia checked her cervical mucus. "I had so much of it," says Nan, "it was coming out of me like chicken soup. I apologized to him for it." "But that's good," he said, "very good." Nan got off the table and went with him into the ultrasound room. Lying on her back on the table, she watched his face as he looked at the screen. "I see three follicles on the right ovary and some others on the left one," he said. "I don't know if they will all have good eggs; some may be immature, or too old. Your ovaries might be all covered over by scar tissue from the laparotomy we did. There's no way of knowing that until we do the laparoscopy." Nan could see how hard he was working to prepare her for disappointment, but she sensed that behind his words he was optimistic. Her fears vanished.

Nan went back to the hotel. She and Todd spent the rest of the day in their room, resting quietly in preparation for the surgery the next day. They ordered dinner in their room. Nan was not to have anything to eat or drink after midnight. At ten, they turned out the light and went to sleep.

An hour later, they were awakened by the hotel fire alarm. They rushed out into the hallway and found it full of people. "We didn't know if this was going to be a Towering Inferno or what. All we wanted to do was get out alive," says Nan. "My laparoscopy was in eight hours. I was supposed to be staying calm and getting a good night's sleep, and here we were walking down eight flights of stairs to get out of the hotel." After milling around outside the hotel for an hour, the guests were notified that it had been a false alarm.

Nan and Todd gratefully went back to their room. They turned on the television and watched "Saturday Night Live" with Rod Stewart to calm themselves down. Nan slept fitfully the rest of the night. She kept having the same dream over and over again. She was shopping at Waldbaum's Drug Store, the one in the shopping mall near Sea Cliff. There were three seven-year-old boys with her, each one of them a carbon copy of Todd, and they were all clamoring for her to buy them something.

7

Laparoscopy
and Transfer

Nan woke up at four forty-five, looked at the clock, and tried to go back to sleep. At five-fifteen, she gave up and got out of bed. She took a shower, got dressed, then woke Todd. The Tiltons arrived at the Surgical Diagnostic Unit of Norfolk General Hospital just at six-thirty. Shari and another in vitro patient, Betsy Hanna, were already there. The women were given wristbands with their names and taken to the preoperative waiting room, where they took off their clothes and put on hospital gowns. Betsy Hanna was going to be first. She had already been through the in vitro procedure three times before, so she was an old hand at it. When Betsy was ready, a nurse walked her down the hall to the operating room.

Nan and Shari were both nervous. They were told they could visit with their husbands for a few minutes, then the nurse came to get Nan. Nan got into a bed in the preop room to wait. While she was waiting, Betsy was brought out of surgery, still unconscious. Now Nan was really nervous. "I was dying," says Nan. "I'd gotten this far. Was I going to make it to the next hurdle?" The operating room nurse, Margaret Whitfield, came to Nan's bedside then to explain to her what was going to happen during the laparoscopy.

The patient is taken to the operating room fully awake, and without any medication. "We don't know the effects of drugs or anesthesia on the eggs," explains Dr. Garcia, "therefore we try to withhold them until the last possible minute." The patient lies down on the operating table and nurses in the operating room prepare her. They put her feet into stirrups, then cover her legs with leg warmers. Another nurse inserts the IV. While the patient is being draped with sterile cloths, the anesthesiologist is getting ready to start the general anesthesia. The patient is then tipped down

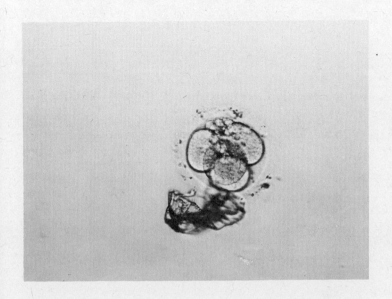

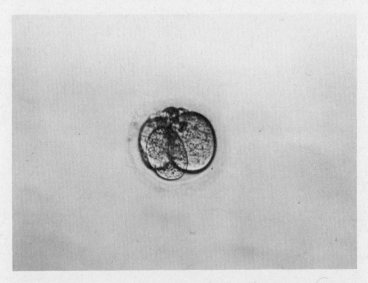

Actual photographs of two of the Tiltons' four embryos at forty-five hours old while still in the laboratory, before being transferred to Nan Tilton's uterus.

Credit: The Howard and Georgeanna Jones Institute for Reproductive Medicine

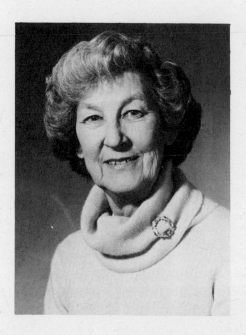

Dr. Georgeanna Seegar Jones, and Dr. Howard W. Jones, Jr., co-founders and co-directors of the first In Vitro Fertilization Clinic in the United States, at the Eastern Virginia Medical School, Norfolk, Virginia.

Credit: Audiovisual Services, Norfolk General Hospital

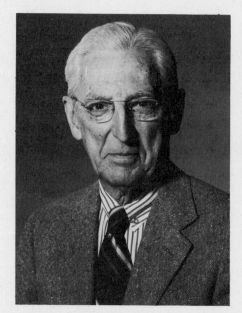

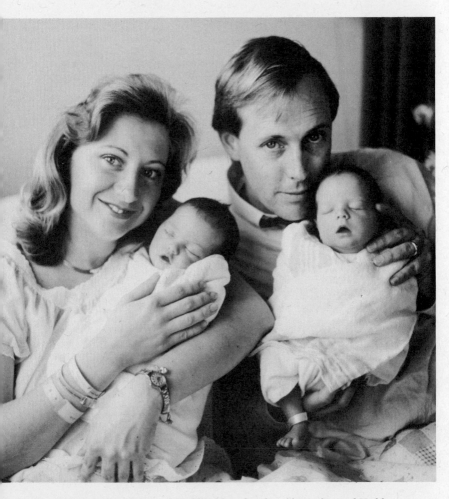

First formal portrait: Nan and Todd holding five-day-old Heather and Todd at North Shore University Hospital.

Credit: Kathryn Abbe

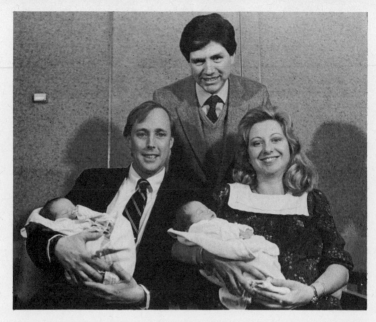

Dr. Jairo E. Garcia of the In Vitro Fertilization Program, Eastern Virginia Medical School, Norfolk, Virginia, with the Tilton family at the babies' debut press conference on March 28, 1983.

Credit: North Shore University Hospital

Nan and Todd leaving the hospital with the babies, March 30, 1983.

Credit: Newsday Photo by Karen Wiles

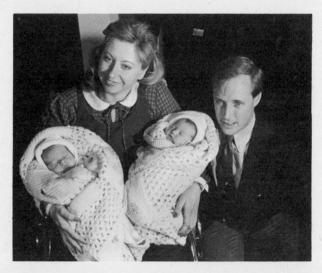

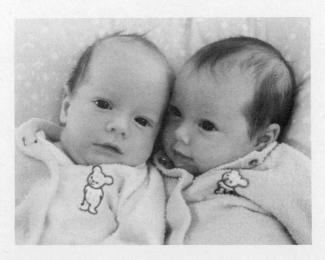

Heather and Todd at home at two weeks old.
Credit: Nan Tilton

The Tilton family at home. The babies are one month old.
Credit: Kathryn Abbe

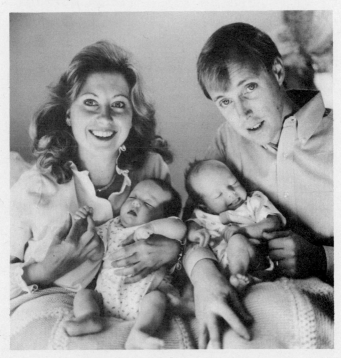

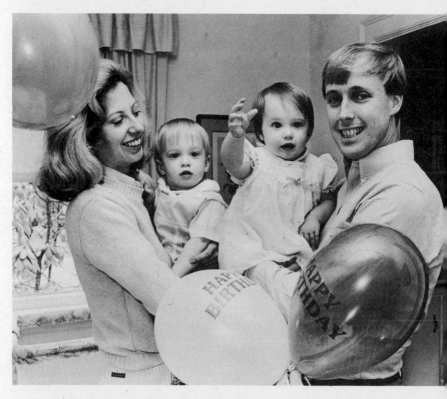

Babies celebrate their first birthday, March 24, 1984.
Credit: Newsday Photo by Bob Luckey

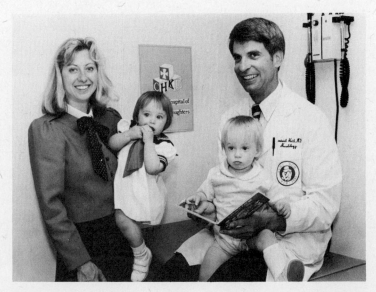

Heather and Todd with Nan, at the babies' first examination by Dr. Frederick H. Wirth at Children's Hospital of the King's Daughters in Norfolk, Virginia, at fourteen months old. Both children were determined to be normal and healthy. Dr. Wirth is conducting the first study of I.V.F. babies.

Credit: Barbara King, Children's Hospital of the King's Daughters

Heather and Todd playing together at eighteen months old.

Credit: Nan Tilton

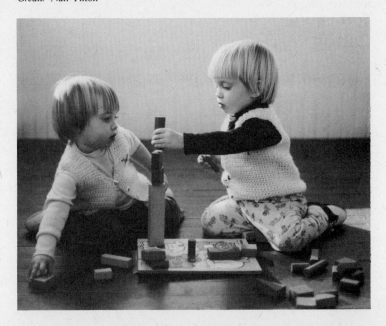

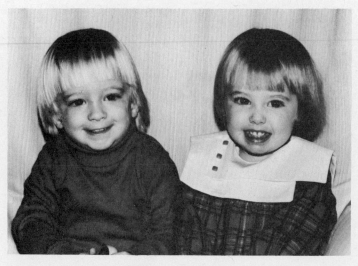

Heather and Todd's second Christmas, December 1984.
Credit: Nan Tilton

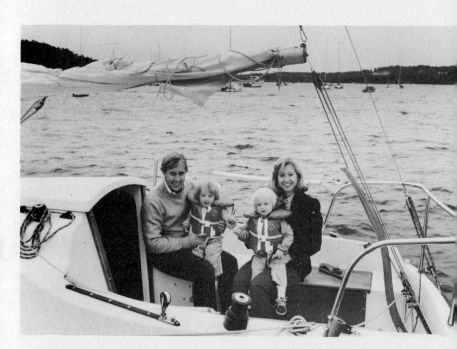

The dream come true: the Tilton family together on their sailboat, fall 1984.
Credit: Kathryn Abbe

to a 45-degree angle, her head down, her legs in the air. This position takes advantage of the force of gravity, allowing the intestines to fall away from the pelvic organs.

When the patient is asleep, the surgeon makes a small incision at the lower edge of the navel. A hollow needle is inserted in the incision and, as mentioned earlier, the abdomen is filled with carbon dioxide gas in order to push the abdominal wall away from the uterus and ovaries. This gives the surgeon room to work. The needle is removed then and the laparoscope inserted. The laparoscope acts as both flashlight and microscope. Through the laparoscope the surgeon can see the ovaries and the developing follicles.

At Norfolk General Hospital, the laparoscope is attached to a small video camera that projects the image that the laparoscope picks up onto two large television screens in the operating room so that everyone on the surgical team can see what the surgeon sees. With the laparoscope, the surgeon looks for follicles on the ovaries. The follicles appear as dark blue, bubble-like protrusions. Inside the follicles are the eggs.

When the surgeon sees that there are indeed follicles on the ovaries, and there is no scar tissue on the ovaries, which would impede the aspiration of the follicles, he makes a second incision and sometimes a third one, lower down on the abdomen. One is for the insertion of an instrument that will hold the ovary still, the other incision is for the needle that will puncture the follicles and aspirate the eggs. At Norfolk, the technique is to make only two incisions.

The needle that aspirates the eggs from the follicles is hollow. At one end is a 45-degree sharpened bevel, the purpose of which is to puncture the follicle so that the egg inside can be aspirated. At the other end of the needle is a plastic test tube into which the egg is aspirated. This is called a collection tube.

The surgeon's first task is to locate all the ripe follicles. To do that, he moves and lifts the ovaries so that he can see them on all sides. When he locates a ripe follicle, he places the needle over it and rotates it gently until the follicle is punctured. Another surgeon standing at his side then aspirates the fluid from the follicle into the collection tube by suction. If the follicle has been successfully punctured, it collapses, much as a blister would collapse when punctured. The egg and the fluid surrounding the egg are now in the collection tube at the other end of the needle. This tube is taken immediately to the laboratory adjoining the operating room by the operating room nurse.

In the laboratory, the embryologist examines the contents of the collection tube under the microscope to confirm that the surgeon has retrieved the egg contained in the follicle he punctured, and to classify the maturity of the egg. The egg is either mature, called a preovulatory oocyte, immature, or postmature, sometimes degenerate. "Usually," says Dr. Garcia, "we get a third of each kind. If the egg is postmature, we try to get a sperm sample from the husband right away and inseminate the egg immediately. But generally these eggs don't fertilize. The degenerate eggs cannot be fertilized. They are dead cells and are discarded."

Immature eggs, however, can be matured in the incubator and have a good chance of fertilizing. "Of all oocytes we classify as immature at aspiration, 83 percent," says Dr. Garcia, "will mature in the laboratory. Out of that group that matures, we will have about a 73 percent fertilization rate. This is very good. It means that we can increase the number of eggs available for fertilization."

The most desirable egg for the purpose of in vitro fertilization and subsequent implantation is the preovulatory, mature egg. Embryologist Lucinda Veeck says, "At Norfolk now, with the combination Pergonal-FSH hormone stimulation, 93 percent of the preovulatory eggs that we retrieve fertilize. This is an improvement over the Pergonal only stimulation protocol. We were getting 86 to 87 percent fertilization rate with Pergonal."

After the embryologist looks at the egg under the microscope, he communicates the status of the egg to the operating room by means of an intercom system. No matter how many times the Norfolk in vitro team has heard the word "preov" come over the intercom, they still break into loud cheers and hearty applause for every mature egg they retrieve.

In July 1982, when Nan Tilton went into the operating room, the most eggs the Norfolk in vitro team had ever gotten from a patient was four, and four was unusual. The usual number of eggs retrieved was two. Only two years later, in June 1984, it was not unusual during egg retrieval to get nine or ten eggs. The difference is in the hormone stimulation protocol used. The average number of eggs being retrieved at Norfolk today is over six.

The Norfolk in vitro team usually gets the first egg within four to five minutes after the patient has been anesthetized. The same puncture and aspiration procedure is repeated for every follicle on both ovaries. The surgeon assigns each follicle a number. A nurse in the operating room records the contents of each follicle, its size, thickness, transparency, aspiration time, volume of fluid aspirated, color, a description of the egg retrieved, and the classification assigned to the egg. This information goes into a computer along with all the other information about each patient and helps the Norfolk in vitro team assess the results of the hormone stimulation protocol used in the current series of patients. By comparing the results of the current cycle of patients with prior groups of patients, and by looking at the responses of one individual patient over two or three previous in vitro attempts, Dr. Georgeanna Jones decides on the general protocol to be used on the next series of in vitro patients, and the individual protocol for each patient who returns for another attempt.

Sometimes the embryology lab cannot find an egg in the fluid aspirated from the follicle and informs the operating room. The surgeon then goes back to irrigate the follicle. He flushes fluid into the follicle, then draws it out again hoping to pull in the recalcitrant egg along with it. When all the existing follicles have been punctured and aspirated, the surgeon returns to each one of them and performs this irrigation procedure to make sure he has gotten the egg from every follicle.

The laparoscopy is now over. The instruments are removed and the carbon dioxide gas is expelled through the incisions. The incisions are closed with a few stitches and covered with Band-Aids. The entire procedure has taken less than half an hour. The patient wakes up in the recovery room and is notified soon after as to how many eggs have been retrieved. The patient stays at the hospital for several hours, until the anesthesia has fully worn off. The patient is given a prescription for tetracycline, an antibiotic which is to be taken for forty-eight hours to prevent infection as a result of the surgery, and then released.

The eggs that have been retrieved are put into an incubator in the laboratory for six hours if they are mature, longer if they are immature. It is time now for the husband to provide the sperm to fertilize the eggs. When the wife goes into surgery, the husband is given two specimen containers. One semen specimen is required a few hours after the laparoscopy for the mature eggs that have been retrieved; the second specimen may be required twenty-four hours or more later if immature eggs have been retrieved. The husband must deliver the semen no longer than thirty minutes after it has been collected. It is important that the semen be kept close to body temperature until it is delivered. "One husband put the semen container on the dashboard of his car to drive over to the hospital," says Dr. Garcia. "It was a very hot day. By the time he got to the laboratory, the sperm were all dead."

When the semen sample arrives in the laboratory, it is washed until the semen plasma has been separated from the sperm. "We spin the sperm in a centrifuge to separate the best part of the sperm, the most motile sperm, from the rest," says Lucinda Veeck. "Then we incubate these sperm for about two hours. At the end of two hours, we put anywhere from 50,000 to 100,000 motile sperm into the petri dish with the wife's egg, and then put the dish back into the incubator."

Seventeen hours later, the embryologist takes this petri dish out of the incubator and looks at it under the microscope. "At that time," says Lucinda Veeck, "we should see two pronuclei, which means the embryo has begun to divide into two cells. This is the earliest sign of fertilization." What has happened during this seventeen hours is that one of the 50,000 to 100,000 sperm in the petri dish has penetrated the outer covering of the egg, called the cumulus, and the outer membrane, called the pellucida, and is united with the egg. The egg and sperm become one cell. Before long, the one cell will begin to divide, forming first two cells, then four, and eight, and so on. "The embryo is put back into the incubator overnight and the next day, we should see under the microscope a conceptus that ranges from two to eight cells."

Meanwhile, the immature eggs that have been retrieved during the laparoscopy have been in the incubator overnight. About 80 percent of them mature during this twenty-four-hour period of incubation. The immature eggs that do mature during incubation are just as likely to fertilize as the mature eggs that have been retrieved. At this point, the husband provides a second semen sample, and the laboratory processes it in the same way.

"Depending on how many fertilized eggs we obtain from these mature and immature eggs," says Dr. Garcia, "we determine when the best time is to transfer them to the patient's uterus. The transfer usually occurs two or three days after laparoscopy. At this time, all of the eggs that have successfully fertilized and divided to the eight-cell stage will be transferred. There is always the possibility that under these conditions twins or triplets will develop. But so far, this has proved to be the exception. The chance of having twins by in vitro fertilization is 8 percent and triplets 2.5 percent. In many more instances, only *one* of the embryos we transfer develops."

The day after the laparoscopy, the patient rests. The second day after laparoscopy, the patient reports to the office at Medical Tower in the morning for a blood test. "We must know for sure that the levels of estrogen are appropriate to receive the embryos in the environment most conducive to their implantation," explains Dr. Garcia. These blood tests will be done every other day for the next two weeks.

Also on the second day after laparoscopy, the patient begins to receive injections of progesterone on a daily basis. If the patient is pregnant, the progesterone injections will be continued daily for seven days, then weekly for the first eighteen weeks of the pregnancy. Progesterone is a hormone produced by the ovaries to prepare the cervix and uterus for fertilization. The purpose of administering progesterone to in vitro patients at this stage is to prevent any disruption of the body's natural luteal phase, the surge of luteinizing hormone that triggers the mature egg to burst from the ovary, which might have been provoked by the aspiration of the follicles. The progesterone injections also help build up the endometrial lining of the uterus in case the embryos that are transferred do implant and pregnancy is achieved.

The more the nurse explained to Nan, the more terrified she became. It was Nan's turn now to get out of the bed and walk down the long hallway to the operating room. On the way there, she passed a conference room. The door was open. Nan couldn't help looking in. "Dr. Howard Jones, Jr., and Dr. Garcia were in there with their heads together," says Nan. "I just knew they were discussing me." She suddenly felt faint and grabbed the nurse's arm for support. "Don't worry," murmured the nurse. "You're going to be all right."

"She was so reassuring," says Nan. "I didn't feel so alone."

In the operating room, a whole battalion of nurses converged on Nan all at once, one fixing her legs in the stirrups, another putting on leg warmers, another starting the IV. "I felt so strange, having all these people touching me." After Nan was in position on the table, a nurse swabbed Betadine, a disinfectant, over her stomach and draped her body with sterile cloths. As they were completing their preparations, Nan's legs started trembling and her teeth began chattering. "I was so embarrassed," says Nan. "I didn't want them to think I was a sissy."

Dr. Acosta came in then and the nurses put the last sterile cloth over Nan's face. "It would have been frightening," says Nan, "except that a minute later I was out."

Nan woke up in the recovery room forty-five minutes later. Todd was sitting next to her bed, and Dr. Acosta had just come into the room. He came right over to her bed. "Mrs. Tilton," he said, "I have very good news for you. The surgery we performed several months ago was a complete success. You healed beautifully. There was absolutely no scarring or adhesions; we could see everything. The ovaries were completely accessible for egg retrieval."

"How many eggs, how many eggs did you get?" asked Nan impatiently. Dr. Acosta leaned down close to her ear and motioned Todd to come nearer. "Mrs. Tilton," he whispered, "we got five eggs."

"Five eggs," says Nan. "I'd never even heard of that many before. No one got five eggs."

"As you know," said Dr. Acosta, "the number of eggs we retrieve is no guarantee that they will all fertilize. We don't want to get your hopes up too high, nor do we want to discourage the other patients unnecessarily. After all, we have achieved a pregnancy with only one embryo transferred. So it's best to keep the number of eggs we retrieved today confidential."

Nan lay back in her bed, her eyes seeking Todd's. They were indeed blessed. She closed her eyes then, as Todd did, to pray. Shari was brought in a few minutes later, still unconscious. She was just coming out of the anesthesia when Dr. Howard Jones, Jr., and Dr. Garcia walked by. Nan overheard their words distinctly. " 'Three out of three,' I heard Dr. Jones say. 'That's the way I like it.' It turned out they'd gotten good eggs from all three of us," says Nan. "Shari and Betsy both had two eggs. I told them I had two eggs too."

When Nan's five eggs were analyzed in the laboratory, two were found to be mature, two were immature, and one was degenerate. The two immature eggs were put into the incubator overnight to ripen, the degenerate egg was discarded. The two mature eggs would be ready for fertilization in six hours. Todd was told to deliver his first semen specimen to "Labor and Delivery" at Norfolk General Hospital at two that afternoon.

Nan and Todd stayed with Betsy and Shari and their husbands in the recovery room until noon. Then they were released. Before they left the hospital, the nurse gave them a set of instructions for the postlaparoscopy phase. Todd was to use one of the specimen jars he had been given for sperm to fertilize the two mature eggs. The other jar was provided should the two immature eggs mature overnight. The Tiltons were told to be at Dr. Garcia's office at ten the next morning.

Back at the hotel, Nan went right to bed. "I felt some soreness in my abdomen. There were two incisions, one in my belly button and a little hole down below. They had closed them with stitches." While Nan was lying in bed, Todd was pacing up and down the room, waiting until one-thirty. "Poor Todd," says Nan. "The pressure was really on him now to fertilize those eggs. There were so many women down there in Norfolk with husbands with normal sperm counts, and in vitro wasn't working for them. We didn't really know if it was possible for my eggs and Todd's sperm to blend to make an embryo. There might be some incompatibility we didn't know about. Or maybe Todd's sperm would make an abnormal baby. Dr. Garcia told me that was impossible; weak sperm aren't strong enough to make a baby. I was afraid for Todd. If he couldn't fertilize the eggs, he would feel so horrible."

Todd felt the pressure but used every bit of his power of positive thinking to get through the next hour. "Nan had to go home pregnant," says Todd, "or she would be a basket case again." At one-thirty, when Todd collected his semen Nan was fast asleep. "I remember lying there in bed thinking I should do something to help reassure Todd," says Nan, "but I couldn't keep my eyes open. My part was over then, I felt, until the transfer."

When Todd had finished, he went over to the bed and told Nan he was leaving for the hospital. "She didn't even hear me," says Todd. Todd had put his specimen jar inside a paper bag. He'd written his name on the side of the bag and the top of the bag, and put his name twice on the specimen jar. "I wasn't taking any chances on its getting mixed up with someone else's sperm," says Todd. The car was already waiting down in front of the hotel, the motor running and the air conditioning going. "I sure didn't want those few sperm I had dying on me on the way over to the hospital." At two o'clock on the dot, Todd delivered his sperm to "Labor and Delivery."

When Todd got back to the hotel, Nan was still sleeping. He ordered dinner brought to their room. Todd had a hearty appetite that night; he ate steak. Nan felt too nauseated to eat. She went right back to sleep and slept deeply all night long. Todd though was awake, wondering about his sperm. "If the eggs didn't fertilize, it would be my fault," says Todd. "Nan had done her job. Could I do mine?"

The next day, Monday, July 12, Nan and Todd were sitting in Room 304 Medical Tower at the appointed time, along with the women getting their daily injections and blood tests. That all seemed like so long ago to Nan. The Tiltons knew they would have to wait until all the pelvics and ultrasounds had been done before they could see Dr. Garcia. "We were so nervous thinking about our eggs over there all alone in the laboratory," says Nan, "wondering if they were fertilizing. . . ." They went out in the hall to wait.

Just then Dr. Georgeanna Jones got off the elevator. "What are you doing here?" she asked the Tiltons sternly. "We're waiting to hear about our eggs," said Todd. "Oh no," she said. "You're not supposed to be here." "But the nurse told us to come at ten this morning," said Todd. "You got the wrong information," said Dr. Jones. "We have a thousand eggs over there in the lab to look at. We don't have time to talk to everyone who comes around asking about theirs. Go back to your hotel room and wait for a telephone call."

As Nan and Todd turned to go, Dr. Jones called them back. "Did they give you two specimen containers?" she asked. Todd nodded, and she disappeared down the hall. "I knew then," said Nan, "that she knew who we were. It made me think there was something good going on with our eggs, or she wouldn't have been so concerned about our having a second specimen container."

Nan and Todd drove back to the hotel, their anxiety making them tense and short with one another. What were they going to do all day, waiting for their telephone call? They couldn't go down to the pool; Nan couldn't concentrate on anything; she wanted Todd to talk to her, but he was reading the newspaper. Fifteen minutes later, the telephone rang. Nan was closest to the phone so she picked it up. "Mrs. Tilton," said Dr. Garcia, "two of your eggs have fertilized, and one more has matured, so we need your husband to do his part again." "Todd, we have two embryos!" Nan shrieked. "He should do it as soon as possible," said Dr. Garcia, "and take the specimen to the hospital, fourth floor, 'Labor and Delivery'; they're waiting for him."

When Nan hung up the phone, Todd was crying. "I'd never ever seen him cry before," says Nan. Seeing his tears, Nan was more moved than she had ever been. He had done it, he had fertilized her eggs. "For four years, doctors had been telling Todd and me that we couldn't make a baby," says Nan, "and we had done it. Together, Todd and I had finally made an embryo." She hugged Todd and together they cried. It was going to be easy this time to get a specimen, Todd thought. His sperm worked.

Nan remembers the sequence of events then as though it had happened yesterday. "We were worried that Todd's sperm count wouldn't have had time to build up in twenty-four hours. When you're trying to get pregnant, the infertility doctors tell you it's important not to have intercourse more than once every four days. Now Todd was having to produce sperm two days in a row."

It was a very hot day. "It was about a hundred degrees out," remembers Nan. "I went down and got the car from the parking lot and brought it around to the front entrance where all those men in safari hats were waiting. I had the air conditioning blasting. Todd came out with the little brown bag in his hand and got into the driver's seat. I held the bag with his sperm in my lap. It reminded me of the times I'd gone to pick up donor sperm for my artificial insemination. But this wasn't some other guy's sperm now that was going to make me pregnant. It was Todd's, my husband's, sperm."

When they got to the hospital, Nan and Todd both went up to the fourth floor to deliver Todd's semen specimen. They stayed to see it safely delivered into the right hands, and then their part was over. For that last half hour, Nan had the sensation that for the first time in the entire in vitro procedure, she was actively participating in the experience. "When you first begin in vitro," says Nan, "you get the hormone shots that make the eggs mature, then you lie on a table while they look at you with the pelvics and ultrasound exams, then you lie on the operating table while they take the eggs out. But driving over to the hospital, taking the sperm to the egg, I was *acting* for the first time. I was physically doing something myself to make a baby."

There was nothing to do now though but wait, again. To pass the time, Nan and Todd drove out to a shopping mall for lunch. Afterward they decided to get hair cuts. They found a unisex hair salon and there they sat, side by side, in front of the mirror, vibrant as though with the afterglow of sexual intimacy, only the baby they had just made was in a laboratory two miles away. As Nan and Todd's golden blond hair dropped on the floor around them, the afterglow burned down and was replaced by a concern for the welfare of those embryos in a petri dish which was not unlike the concern of parents for a newborn infant. Were they being kept warm enough? thought Nan. Was someone watching them? "I wanted to be over there with them."

Nan wanted to go back to the hotel to be within calling range if something should happen, so they went back. They didn't have to be at Medical Tower or anywhere else that day, so they put on their bathing suits. Nan had brought a one-piece bathing suit especially for her postlaparoscopy pool days, to cover the stitches. "That's how you could tell which girls had had their surgery," says Nan. They told the hotel clerk to forward their phone calls to the pool area, and went downstairs.

As soon as the Tiltons got to the pool, they were surrounded by the other in vitro patients. How many eggs? How many fertilized? Everyone wanted to know. Nan told them two. They learned that another woman at the pool had had three eggs. "She was walking around the place like a peacock," says Nan. When it came time for this woman's transfer, however, only one egg had fertilized.

Nan could tell too which women had had their transfers. "The husbands were waiting on them, bringing them sodas, moving their lounge chairs to the right spot. The husbands wouldn't let the women bend over or lift anything, because, you see, after the transfer the women considered themselves pregnant."

Todd sat down next to Bob Nelson to compare notes. "He'd written his name all over the specimen jar too," says Todd. Todd had the first drink he'd had in two weeks. "Boy, did it taste good," he says. "I was celebrating. My job was done."

When Nan and Todd went back up to their room two hours later, Dr. Garcia called to tell them to be in his office at ten the next morning. "We will know by then if the other two eggs have fertilized." Nan was so excited she didn't know what to do with herself. "I couldn't imagine how I was going to get through the next eighteen hours," says Nan.

She and Todd decided to go up to the Nelsons' room to see Andrea. She had had two embryos transferred two days before. They found her lying on her stomach on the bed, as per Dr. Garcia's instructions. She wanted to be waited on.

"I feel like chicken for dinner tonight," Andrea said. "Get me chicken."

Bob and Todd went out to get the food and Nan stayed with Andrea. It seemed like hours before the men came back. By that time, Nan was tired and almost sick with hunger. All she was thinking about were her eggs over in the laboratory, and when she was going to have them put back inside her. "The transfer was the good part," says Nan. "The transfer made you pregnant. I couldn't wait." The Tiltons ate quickly, then went to their room and went to bed.

At ten the next morning, July 13, the Tiltons reported to the office at Medical Tower. The nurse took Nan's blood, then she went back to the waiting room, where Shari and her husband were waiting to hear about their eggs too. Dr. Garcia appeared in the doorway. "Who wants to be first?" he said. "I have good news for everybody. Mrs. Tilton?" Nan and Todd followed Dr. Garcia into his office and sat down. Dr. Garcia went around to his side of the desk, and instead of his usually severe expression, he was smiling. "As you know," he said, "your first two eggs fertilized and divided. I am pleased to tell you that the other two eggs have also matured and fertilized. You have four embryos. This is only the second time we at Norfolk will be implanting four embryos."

Nan knew who the other patient with four embryos had been. It was a woman who had been an in vitro patient when Nan was in Norfolk for her diagnostic screening laparoscopy. She had had four embryos transferred and she had not gotten pregnant.

"Our policy here at Norfolk," Dr. Garcia continued, "is that we transfer all the embryos that develop. This means that the chances now of Mrs. Tilton getting pregnant are close to 50 percent."

After everything that Nan and Todd had been through, all the doctors who had told them they would never be able to have a baby, they had *never* had odds like that, ever. "We came to Norfolk thinking we had less of a chance than other people because of my surgery, which might have scarred over the ovaries, and because of Todd's low sperm count," says Nan. "We always felt like we were in the back of the pack, running hard to catch up. Now here we were, the lucky ones."

The practice of telling a patient *before* transfer how many embryos will be implanted has been changed since Nan Tilton was in Norfolk. It is now the practice at the EVMS VIP Program to wait until *after* the transfer. "So many things can happen to the embryos," says Dr. Howard Jones, Jr. "We found ourselves having to tell patients at the transfer that we were going to implant fewer embryos than we'd told them earlier. Therefore, to spare our patients disappointment, we have changed our policy."

Dr. Garcia told the Tiltons to be at the hospital that afternoon at two o'clock on the dot for their transfer.

The embryo transfer is a relatively simple procedure. The embryos are transferred by catheter directly into the patient's uterus. No anesthesia is required for this procedure. At the Norfolk VIP Program, the position they prefer the patient to take for the transfer is the knee-chest position. The patient kneels on the operating table, her bottom in the air, her chest and right cheek pressed down on the table. The doctor inserts a speculum to open the vagina, checks the cervix to be sure it is free of infection, then wipes away the cervical mucus so that the opening of the cervix is clearly visible.

When the patient is in position, Lucinda Veeck in the laboratory next door loads the embryos into a very fine flexible Teflon catheter that has a syringe at one end. Into the catheter she puts first a small quantity of the culture medium in which the embryos have been incubating, then an air space, then the embryos in their culture medium, another air space, and finally another layer of culture medium as a buffer. To do this very delicate work, Lucinda Veeck does not wear sterile gloves; nor does the doctor wear gloves to do the transfer. EVMS has done a thorough quality control analysis on all the instruments and substances which might come into contact with the embryos, in experiments using mouse embryos. Researchers have found that the talcum powder that lines surgical gloves is extremely toxic to embryos, as is alcohol. Therefore it is imperative that both be eliminated from this phase of the in vitro procedure.

When the embryos are loaded, Lucinda Veeck takes the catheter into the operating room and slides it into a metal guide. The purpose of the guide is to allow the catheter just the right degree of penetration into the uterus. Mrs. Veeck hands the apparatus to the doctor and he inserts the guide holding the catheter into the uterus, right up to the cervix, then slides the catheter through the opening of the cervix deep into the uterus. The doctor wears a light on his head as miners do, in order to be able to see clearly into the vagina. The embryos are then expelled into the uterus by means of the syringe at the end. The patient barely feels it.

When the transfer has been completed, Mrs. Veeck takes the empty catheter back to the laboratory and examines it to be sure that the embryos have not been left inside. The patient then moves down slowly onto her stomach and remains in that position without moving for four hours. At the end of four hours, the patient goes home, but she must take it easy for the next twenty-four hours, no strenuous activity. Patients must not climb stairs for two days afterward.

When the Tiltons came out of Dr. Garcia's office, it was the Johnsons' turn. They went in, and Nan and Todd waited for them. Shari and her husband came out twenty minutes later and Shari was in tears. Nan jumped up, instinctively expecting the worst. "Only one of my eggs fertilized," sobbed Shari. Nan was shocked. "Here we were with four embryos," says Nan; "our good fortune was sort of overwhelming. It made me feel guilty almost, and afraid. I didn't see how we could have been so lucky that it worked for us, when it wasn't working for so many other couples." The four of them decided to go out to breakfast together, but no one had any appetite. Shari was so upset that it made all four of them edgy.

On the way back to the hotel, it started raining. It began as any summer rainstorm, but by the time Nan and Todd got up to their room, the rain was coming down in torrents. From the window they could see that the streets were flooding. "What if after all this we can't get to the hospital?" said Nan. She lay down on the bed with a magazine and Todd worked on some things he'd brought from the office. They decided to leave the hotel in plenty of time to get to the hospital. Even so, they were fifteen minutes late. Nan was frantic. As soon as Todd pulled up to the entrance, she dashed out of the car and ran in to tell the receptionist on the main floor to call Dr. Garcia to tell him they were on their way up to the fourth floor. "You can't go up there," said the receptionist. "No one's allowed past the fire doors. The hospital has been hit by lightning. There's no electricity." "We have to go upstairs," yelled Nan. "Our embryos are being transferred." Todd arrived then. He didn't pay any attention to the receptionist. He grabbed Nan by the hand and pulled her toward the stairway. "I was going to get Nan to the fourth floor if it killed me," says Todd. Just then the elevator door opened. The receptionist let them go. "I guess they've turned on the generators," she said to the closing elevator door.

When they got to the fourth floor, Todd went to the waiting room and Nan rushed to the preop room, where she changed into a hospital gown. Debbie Perry, the circulating nurse, walked her down to the operating room. There, outside the door, leaning casually against the wall, wearing his hospital greens, his mask dangling around his neck, Dr. Garcia was waiting for Nan, smiling. Nan thought he was going to be upset with her for being late, but he seemed oblivious to her tardiness.

"How do you feel?" he asked her. "Fine," said Nan uncertainly, wondering what was happening. Dr. Garcia leaned down. "I'm ready to write your name in the book I keep for the patients who get pregnant," he said. "What?" said Nan. He smiled and said nothing more. Nan couldn't believe this was the same Dr. Garcia who was always so careful not to be encouraging. "Here he was," says Nan, "practically assuring me I was going to get pregnant. At that moment I felt very close to him."

Dr. Garcia stood back to let Nan go into the operating room first, then he followed her in. The nurses took her to the operating table and got her into position, her head turned to the side and her cheek resting on the table, her bottom in the air. "Ready," said the nurse. Dr. Garcia went over to the table then and notified the laboratory over the intercom that he was ready. "Loading," came the voice of Lucinda Veeck. It made Nan think of a pinball machine: "All those little silver balls lined up in the starting channel, all four of the embryos lined up, then you pull back the plunger and give it a zap and all the balls go flying."

Suddenly Dr. Garcia turned to the nurse and said, "Do you have the flashlight?" She lifted it in the air to show him she had it in her hand. "The lights went out during Betsy Hanna's transfer," she told Nan. Nan was horrified. "I could imagine all my embryos spilling onto the floor . . ." At that moment, the door to the laboratory opened and Lucinda

Veeck came out holding the catheter with Nan and Todd's four embryos, and handed it to Dr. Garcia. Nan didn't feel anything more than a slight pressure, and it was over. "A beautiful transfer," said Margaret. She told Nan to lie down slowly on her stomach and then went to get a stretcher. She and Debbie lifted Nan carefully onto the stretcher, then over the loudspeaker from the laboratory came the words "All clear." "Now I knew for sure those four embryos were safe inside me," says Nan, "where they should be, with Mama. I was taking care of them now, not the lab technicians."

As Margaret wheeled Nan out of the room, the stretcher bumped into the doorjamb. Nan screamed, grabbing Margaret's arm. "It's all right," said Margaret. "They didn't pop out." She wheeled Nan down the hall to the recovery room. Betsy Hanna and Shari and her husband were already there. The women barely lifted their heads to greet Nan, so wary were they of moving even one wrong muscle and losing the embryos that had just been put inside them. Todd arrived soon after. He was getting a chair to put beside Nan's bed when Dr. Garcia, his expression grave, appeared in the doorway and asked Todd to step out in the hall for a moment. Nan and Todd exchanged looks of apprehension, then Todd followed him out into the hall.

"Mr. Tilton," said Dr. Garcia, "we have transferred four embryos. I would be very surprised if Mrs. Tilton did not get pregnant. I've done everything I can do for you. Now it is up to God." "If ever I felt Someone was watching over us, guiding us," says Todd, "I knew it with absolute certainty at that moment."

Todd went back into the recovery room to reassure Nan that everything was fine. He had to speak in a low voice. The other couples still did not know that Nan had had four embryos transferred.

The women had to lie there now in that room, on their stomachs, for four hours. There was a television and magazines, but Nan couldn't concentrate. She felt a need to share her happiness, with the other women as well as with Todd. "Shari and I were both weepy," says Nan. "We were *pregnant.* Do you realize how long we all had been trying to get to this point? Even if we all three got our periods in two weeks, we could still say we had been pregnant. I realized that this might be the only chance I ever had in my life to be pregnant."

Only Betsy Hanna was nonchalant about the whole thing. She'd been through it three times before and it hadn't worked. "She knew this wasn't the whole ball game," says Nan. "She could have brought us crashing down if we'd let her. Her husband wasn't even there. He had his suitcase there with him in the recovery room and left to catch a plane as soon as Betsy was brought in."

Nan had been lying in her bed for about half an hour. She and Todd had already been through the story of Nan's transfer several times. The time was dragging interminably. It was really hard to stay still on your stomach for a long time, but Nan was going to follow instructions to the letter. All of a sudden, Nan felt a puddle of liquid ooze out between her legs. "I was in absolute shock," says Nan. "Todd," she said, "my embryos just fell out." Todd leaped out of his chair. "Nan's embryos just fell out," yelled Todd. He rushed out in the hall to find a nurse. Betsy Hanna looked up from her magazine. "Nan, it's all right," she said. "It's not the embryos. That always happens after the transfer."

Nan was not reassured. "I'm not listening to Betsy Hanna about this," said Nan. "I want to know *exactly* what's happening." Just then Dr. Georgeanna Jones put her head in the door. "Hello," she said. "How's everybody in here?" "I just had a pool of liquid come out of me," she said. "What's happening to my embryos?" Dr. Jones came in to pat Nan's head. "You're all right, dear," she said. "It's the liquid we used for the transfer. Your embryos are safe and sound in your uterus. That's why we have you lie on your stomach, so that the uterus is tilted down; they can't come out."

But even Dr. Jones could not fully persuade Nan that her four embryos weren't lying there on the sheet between her legs. "I think all the pressure was finally catching up to me," says Nan. "A lot of the forty-six women who were in our series were going home without getting pregnant, only Maria and one other woman had gotten pregnant. It began to seem to me that in vitro wasn't working. What was I going to say when it didn't work for me? 'My embryos fell out?' Was that going to be the reason *I* didn't get pregnant?"

Todd tried to reason with Nan. "She was really going off the deep end," says Todd. "She'd been steeling her nerves to get through the whole thing, then when everything was over, all her anxieties just blew up, and she fixated on that stuff oozing out of her." Todd just kept repeating what Dr. Jones had said, and gradually Nan began to relax. It was the television that finally succeeded in distracting her. The women had decided to watch *"All in the Family."* Ironically, the episode they watched that day was the one in which Gloria was having her baby. Every one of the women in the room felt it to be a good omen. "It was so exciting," says Nan, "thinking that it might actually happen to us."

At the end of the four hours, Nan got up and very carefully got dressed, putting on everything over her head, rather than lifting her legs. She was taken down to the main lobby in a wheelchair. Todd had the car waiting and they drove back to the hotel. The rain had subsided by then. As slowly as she could, Nan walked through the hotel lobby to the elevators. As soon as she was in the room, she lay down gingerly on her stomach again and fell fast asleep. She dreamed she had three three-year-olds running off in three directions all at once and she couldn't catch any of them. "I felt as though I had three babies, but they could all just as easily vanish right before my eyes" was Nan's interpretation of the dream.

The next morning, July 14, at ten, Nan and Todd Tilton reported to Room 304 Medical Tower for Nan's blood test and her first injection of progesterone. The progesterone injections would continue every day and the blood tests every other day for the next ten to fourteen days. If at that time the presence of HCG in the blood was detected, then pregnancy had been achieved, and the progesterone injections would continue to be administered on a daily basis for another week, and then once a week for the first eighteen weeks of the pregnancy. If the patient was not pregnant, the progesterone injections would be discontinued, and the woman would get her period.

For any woman undergoing in vitro fertilization, this ten-to-fourteen day wait to find out if she is pregnant is interminable. When the Tiltons were going through the in vitro procedure, the policy at the EVMS Vital Initiation of Pregnancy Program was to keep the women in Norfolk during this phase. This is no longer their practice. "We are pretty sure now," says Dr. Howard Jones, Jr., "that if the embryos are going to implant in the uterus, they will implant during those first four hours." But there is also a psychological explanation for the change in policy. "It was too difficult for the women," says Dr. Garcia. "There were too many tensions for them all together. We have found they do much better waiting these two weeks at home. And it sure saves our patients a lot of money on room and board."

Today, patients at Norfolk are each given a Styrofoam box on the day after transfer. Inside the box are enough doses of progesterone for daily injections, and enough test tubes for blood samples which are to be drawn every other day for thirteen days. If they wish, patients can administer the progesterone injections themselves. Doris teaches the patients or their husbands how to give the shots. The blood, however, must be drawn by a professional. The women keep the samples chilled in the refrigerator until the thirteenth day and then mail them all together in the Styrofoam chest, packed in dry ice, by Federal Express so that they arrive in Norfolk twenty-four hours later. The lab in Norfolk runs pregnancy tests on the thirteenth day after transfer. The patients are notified by telephone if they are pregnant or not.

For Nan and Todd Tilton, the waiting was just beginning. Todd flew home to New York the next morning early so that he could be in the office first thing. Five hours later, Nan's mother arrived. "I was lucky to have someone with me," says Nan. "A lot of the women were waiting all alone." Nan's mother took charge of Nan's nest-sitting for the next four days, going out for food and supplies, changing the channel on the television, tucking and smoothing Nan's sheets. No one had told Nan that she had to spend the next two weeks in bed, but Nan decided that if four hours lying on your stomach helped the embryos implant, then ten days of lying in bed would be even better. "I didn't want to have to say someday that it might have worked if only I'd done such and such," says Nan. "I was going to do everything I could do, just like Todd and I had done up until then, to make sure in vitro worked for us."

Andrea Nelson often spent the day in the other bed in Nan's room, and Nan's mother took care of her too. The women were surprised at how relieved they felt not to have their husbands around. "Todd would have been crawling the walls," says Nan. "There's not enough for the men to do here. You feel like you have to entertain them." Another woman who has been down to Norfolk for three in vitro attempts says, "After the men have run a few errands, taken the laundry and picked it up, they sit down in front of the TV and that's it. They're no help at all. This is the women's time. It's fun to just sit around and talk and not have to go somewhere and do something all the time."

Nan's days were lazy and interminably long—shots, breakfast out, back to bed and TV, lunch in the room, then to the pool until nap time, and in the evening, dinner out with the women. In the privacy of her room, Nan took out the book she had brought with her, Lennart Nilsson's *A Child Is Born*, published by Dell in 1966. With photographs taken inside the womb, photographer Nilsson documents the stages of the developing embryo. Every day Nan could look at the book and see what those embryos inside her looked like—at twenty-four hours old, forty-eight hours old, three days.

The tension of waiting reached its peak every morning at Medical Tower when the women found out who was going home that day, not pregnant. As the days went by, the ducks were going down. Nan kept a list of the women in her series: Judy—no, Marianne—no, blond girl—no, little blond-haired girl—no, short-haired girl—no, skinny girl—no, girl with red-haired husband—no, Sue Lane—yes. "She was the only one besides Maria who had gotten pregnant," says Nan.

The tension dissipated then gradually built up throughout the day until dinner when the competition among the women was unspoken but fierce. The uncertainty haunted the women's dreams. Their life in Norfolk was such a powerful reality that it was easy for the women to forget they had another life somewhere else. This was all there was, waiting to find out if they were pregnant.

Two days after Nan's transfer, Andrea Nelson, unable to take the strain of waiting, went home. Her own gynecologist would give her the progesterone shots and take blood samples. Shari too was cracking under the strain. "You really do need nerves of steel to go through in vitro fertilization," says Nan. She had no intention of leaving Norfolk until the end.

Dr. Garcia has observed that the in vitro patients are an astonishing group of people. "Their hope and faith are endless," he says. "This is an important attitude to have during the in vitro process. I am not a psychologist, nor a psychiatrist, but I have seen it very clearly; there is no doubt that a positive attitude helps in vitro to work. Occasionally, we do have patients, of course, who are nervous wrecks. But their anxiety is not based on fear. They are not afraid of the surgery. They have had laparoscopies before. It is because they have been disappointed so many times in their lives. They've had ectopic pregnancies and miscarriages, operations, and they don't want to hear again that they are not pregnant. We have seen these patients conceive by in vitro fertilization.

"But we do have patients," says Dr. Garcia, "who come with very negative attitudes. This makes our work more difficult. I have succeeded in turning many of them around by being firm with them, telling them quite clearly that unless they changed their attitude, they would not get pregnant. I have seen some patients who did not want to have anything to do with the other patients. They wanted to stay by themselves and not integrate with the group. I tell them that this is not normal. They are wasting time and money to come here. I have seen these patients change as they come back to Norfolk for another try. Gradually they start making friends with the other women and they finally conceive."

Dr. Garcia has also seen another quality in in vitro patients. "In some very rare cases," he says, his voice hushed, "I have seen something special, something I can't explain. There is a predisposition, a certain kind of perspective that makes me feel this patient is going to be successful. There is nothing scientific about this feeling at all. I told Dr. Howard Jones that I was concerned because I was developing intuition. But most of the time when I have these feelings I am right. I felt this right away when I met Mrs. Tilton."

As the days went by, Nan watched the women begin to prepare themselves for disappointment. Subtly the women's conversations began to shift to the future. "Everyone was making plans for when they'd come back and try it again. They'd say, 'Let's all come back for the winter session.' " But Nan wouldn't commit herself to any such plans. She hadn't finished yet what she'd come down to Norfolk to do.

One night near the end of the waiting, Nan came back to her room and as she put her keys down on the bureau, she drank in the image of her and Todd holding their godchild in the photograph taped to the mirror. In a flash the image that had always been an inspiration was transformed; it seemed now to be a rebuke, a charade. Nan, for the first time, was afraid. Alone in her room that night, Nan Tilton made a pact with God. "If I have a child," she said, "oh, please, God, I promise to be charitable to other people for the rest of my life."

Pregnancy
and Birth

On Thursday July 22, 1982, nine days after her transfer, Nan Tilton woke up at five-thirty in the morning with cramps. As she lay there in bed, she tried desperately to make a distinction between the cramps she was feeling then and the cramps she had when she was getting her period. "They weren't painful the way menstrual cramps were," says Nan. "They would subside and almost feel good for a moment." In three hours, she would have the blood test that would determine without a doubt whether she were pregnant or not. Nan lay absolutely still and prayed.

At seven the telephone rang. It was Shari. "She was crying so hard I could barely understand her," says Nan. She wanted Nan to meet her down in the lobby and go over to Medical Tower together for their pregnancy tests. Nan got out of bed and went to take a shower. In the bathroom, Nan noticed she had a sticky white discharge. "I'd never had that before," says Nan, her excitement mounting. "I'd read in one of the books I'd brought along that this discharge was a sign of pregnancy." Nan could feel herself about to explode with excitement.

At Medical Tower, Nan went in first to have her blood test. When it was Shari's turn, she was so close to hysteria that Nan took her downstairs and walked her around outside the building for a while to calm her down. "I didn't want her in the waiting room, scaring all the other girls who were new," says Nan. When Shari had stopped crying, they went back up to the office, and Shari had her blood test. Then they both got their progesterone injections. Jan Coleridge told them to come back to the office at four for the results. What could they possibly do for the next six hours?

Nan and Shari got in the car and went back to the hotel to pick up Nan's brother Ronnie so that they could all go out for breakfast. Ronnie had replaced Nan's mother as her companion in Norfolk. "He'd been through his wife's pregnancy," says Nan, "so he knew what being pregnant was like. Every time I felt something I asked him about it. 'Oh, yeah,' he'd say. "Jeanette had those pains for nine months,' and I got really excited." If Nan expressed doubts, he'd say, "You don't know it didn't work until the doctor tells you. Until then, just assume that it worked."

At breakfast, Shari was still crying. Ronnie gave her the same pep talk he gave Nan, and she seemed to feel a little better. The rest of the day was interminable. Nan and Ronnie went down to the pool for a while. One of the in vitro women was boasting to the others that she had had three embryos transferred. "That's when I told everyone I'd had four transferred," says Nan. "I didn't want them to be surprised when they heard I'd gotten pregnant. I was really that optimistic."

While Nan and her brother were out at the pool, Shari was inside in the hotel lobby, running from one pay phone to another, calling Dr. Garcia, her husband, and the airlines to make reservations for a flight home. "First she told Dr. Garcia she didn't want to be in Norfolk to find out if she were pregnant or not. She wanted to fly home immediately to be with her husband. Then she changed her mind and called them all back again. She was on the telephone the whole day. It was terrible to see."

After lunch at the pool, Nan and Ronnie went up to the room and watched television for a while. Then they took the car to the garage to have it checked over for the trip back to New York. Their plan was, if Nan was not pregnant, she and Ronnie would go back to the hotel, throw all their stuff into the car, and go. If Nan was pregnant, she would fly home that afternoon and Ronnie would drive the car home. They put oil and water in the car, filled the tires. It still wasn't four o'clock. They drove over to Medical Tower anyway and then had a soda in the drugstore in the lobby to kill some more time. Nan decided they should go up to the waiting room anyway.

The office was empty, except for two new girls waiting for their afternoon shots. Nan could hardly remember when she'd been a new girl. It was a lifetime ago. The door to the hallway opened and Dr. Garcia came in. He saw Nan and smiled but kept right on going through the waiting room to his office. He came back out again a few minutes later and stood there in the doorway. "Mrs. Tilton?" he said. It was still half an hour until four. "Come with me." Nan got up and followed him into the office area. He carefully closed the door to the waiting room behind her. "Mrs. Tilton," he whispered, "you're pregnant." Nan threw her arms around his neck and hung onto him, hard. "I knew it, I knew it," she chanted, the tears choking her throat. "How did you know?" Dr. Garcia asked. "I could feel it," said Nan. He said, "You can't feel it yet." Of course, Nan hadn't known for certain she was pregnant. She'd worked for it, prayed for it . . . When Nan finally let go of Dr. Garcia, she turned around and there in the hallway was the entire staff of the EVMS VIP Program waiting to congratulate her. "Thank you, thank you," wept Nan, "for making my dream come true."

Nan Tilton's pregnancy was the twenty-third pregnancy at Eastern Virginia Medical School. This meant that by the end of Series V in August 1982, the pregnancy rate at the Norfolk clinic was still 13 percent. Other women too found out that day whether they were pregnant or not. Shari Johnson did not get pregnant. Andrea Nelson did. She was informed by Dr. Garcia by telephone. Seven of the forty-six women in Series V achieved pregnancy.

The news of Nan's pregnancy spread like wildfire among the clinic patients. A woman who had just been told for the third time that in vitro fertilization had not worked for her walked right out of the office where she had received the news to Nan in the waiting room. With tears in her eyes, she embraced Nan and said, "I'm so glad it worked for you." "The strength of that woman," marvels Nan.

Nan rushed downstairs to the lobby to call Todd. She told the operator it was an emergency. All over Marine Midland Bank in New York, people were looking for Todd Tilton. He was found and a telephone thrust into his hand. "The first week of April," said Nan, "you'll be a father," and all the employees of Marine Midland within earshot knew it then too. Nan heard them cheering.

Nan went back upstairs then to wait for the last time in the room where she had waited so long to hear she was pregnant. When Dr. Garcia finished with the other in vitro patients, he gave her instructions for going home.

When a patient becomes pregnant by in vitro fertilization, she is sent home and, for the duration of the pregnancy and birth, she is to be under the care of her own obstetrician. The VIP Program requires only that the obstetrician be a member of a group practice equipped to handle high-risk pregnancies, and be affiliated with a Level Three hospital. A Level Three hospital is a hospital that includes neonatal high-risk services. This requirement was established only as a precaution, should a complication develop during the pregnancy. There is no medical reason, however, for an in vitro pregnancy to be treated any differently than a pregnancy achieved in vivo.

The patient's obstetrician must contact EVMS at the beginning of the pregnancy for instructions. The doctor is instructed to send a blood sample to Norfolk the week after pregnancy has been determined, and to continue the daily injections of progesterone for seven days. Then the doctor will administer weekly injections of a long-acting progesterone called Delalutin for a period of eighteen weeks to prevent miscarriage. In 1982, patients were required to send a sample of their blood, packed in dry ice, via Federal Express to Norfolk once a month for five months for research purposes. It is no longer necessary to do that. The birth is to be by vaginal delivery, unless otherwise indicated by individual circumstances. Eight to ten weeks from the patient's last menstrual period, an ultrasound examination should be made by the obstetrician to monitor the progress of the pregnancy. Amniocentesis is not necessary unless maternal age or past medical history requires it.

The only instruction the patient is given is to avoid alcohol in her diet, and smoking is prohibited. As for sexual intercourse, there are no restrictions for the entire nine months of pregnancy.

If pregnancy is not achieved by in vitro fertilization, patients are instructed to stop the injections of progesterone and their menstrual period will come within a few days. They are encouraged to come back to the VIP Program and try again, but no sooner than two months after the previous in vitro attempt. "It is important that all the anesthesia be eliminated from the body," says Dr. Garcia, "and the liver has time to recover from the medication."

There is no limit to the number of times a couple can try in vitro fertilization. Every time the individual patient attempts in vitro fertilization, the chances of her getting pregnant are the same. The statistical probability that an individual patient will achieve pregnancy does not increase with each successive attempt. If the patient comes back often enough, the statistics show that she eventually will get pregnant. There are several women who have tried nine or ten times. "We have eight patients who have come seven times, and seven of them got pregnant," says Dr. Garcia.

The Norfolk in vitro team is quite glad when a couple decides to return. "We already know so much about them," says Dr. Garcia. "We're not starting with a blank slate. We have a much better idea each time they come, what we can do to try and help them get pregnant." When a woman returns for another in vitro attempt, the VIP team gets together to analyze her patterns of response to the hormone stimulation she was given in the past, and will make modifications in the protocol for her next attempt. "If a woman gets pregnant and miscarries in the first trimester, then we would probably repeat the same stimulation program, but increase her dose of progesterone after the transfer, which might help the embryos implant," says Dr. Garcia. If, as in the case of a patient recently treated for the third time at Norfolk and canceled because follicles had failed to develop at all, even after three different hormone stimulation protocols, the Norfolk team will try administering the hormones on a different schedule, a schedule that is determined by a more closely monitored observation of the patient's response.

Nan flew home to Sea Cliff that night. Todd, and Nan's mother and stepfather, were at the airport to meet her. She moved very slowly. "I felt like I was carrying precious jewels inside of me," says Nan. The very next morning, as soon as she got up, she called Dr. Schachter to make an appointment. She wasn't sure yet she wanted to use Schachter as her obstetrician, but she had to get progesterone shots every day that first week and she had to have somebody give them to her. Dr. Schachter could not see Nan until Wednesday, July 28, five days later, so Nan called her internist and asked him if he could give her the shots until then. The internist arranged for a visiting nurse to give Nan the injections.

On Wednesday, Nan went to her appointment with Dr. Schachter. The office was full. There were several pregnant women in the waiting room and Nan reacted instinctively with the hostility she had long felt toward pregnant women; then her heart leaped with the realization that she no longer had to be jealous of pregnant women. "I was pregnant too," says Nan. She was horrified to see some of the women smoking. "I didn't want to be in the same room with them, breathing that smoke," says Nan, so she went outside to wait.

Nan was finally admitted to the examining room. She had been sitting on the table for fifteen minutes, waiting for Dr. Schachter, when her nurse came in and told Nan she needed that room for someone else, and Nan would have to go to another room. "It was such a contrast," says Nan, "to the way the doctors in Norfolk treated their patients. I'd forgotten that this was the way most doctors were."

Dr. Schachter finally came in. "After all that had happened," says Nan, "the artificial inseminations she did for me, the tube test, her referring us to Dr. Jones, she knew how hard we'd tried to have a baby, and how much the odds were against us . . . She came over to me on the table and patted me on the head. 'So, we're having a baby,' she said. I couldn't believe it. Even as a professional, she should have been more interested in what I'd just been through. But nothing, no excitement, no celebration. She didn't even say, 'That's wonderful.' " Nan decided then that she was going to find another obstetrician. Dr. Schachter gave Nan her injection that day and they made an appointment for the following week. Nan had no intention of keeping it.

Nan knew exactly the obstetrician she wanted. It was Dr. Paul Mazzarella, an ob/gyn in Manhasset. He was associated with a group practice headed by Dr. Arnold Fenton that was affiliated with North Shore University Hospital, a Level Three hospital. Nan knew about him because he had saved a friend's baby in the seventh month of pregnancy. At the first sign of high blood pressure, he began to monitor her blood pressure daily. That was the kind of care Nan wanted, nothing less than around-the-clock dedication.

The next day Nan called Dr. Mazzarella's office to make an appointment. "The doctor has no appointments open until the end of August," said the receptionist. "Tell Dr. Mazzarella that I'm pregnant by in vitro fertilization," said Nan, "and I want him to be my obstetrician." "You mean pregnant by artificial insemination," said the receptionist. Nan found in the months to come that this would be the common reaction to her pregnancy. ("People didn't understand what in vitro fertilization was," says Nan, "even medical people. They kept telling me it was artificial insemination.") "Not artificial insemination," said Nan, "in vitro fertilization . . ." There was silence on the other end of the phone. "A testtube baby," said Nan. "Oh," exclaimed the receptionist, "just a minute." When she came back on the line, she told Nan that Dr. Mazzarella was busy at the moment, but he'd like to talk to her and would call her back.

Five minutes later, the phone rang and it was Dr. Mazzarella. "I understand you are pregnant by in vitro fertilization," he said. "Isn't that wonderful! Would you like to come in today?" Nan melted. "I knew this was the doctor for me," she says. "Is five o'clock all right?" asked Dr. Mazzarella. "I'll be there," said Nan.

That afternoon before her appointment Nan wrote out a list of the questions she had for the doctor who was going to successfully bring her pregnancy to term. She wanted 100 percent commitment to this pregnancy, and she wanted Dr. Mazzarella to know it.

Dr. Mazzarella's office was on the second floor of a professional building in Manhasset, almost across the street from North Shore University Hospital. The waiting room was very large, big enough to accommodate the patients of all six doctors who shared the practice. Two receptionists sat behind a glass enclosed window to direct patients, answer questions, schedule appointments, and take payments when the visits concluded. It looked like a high-powered, well-organized but impersonal operation.

On the dot of five the receptionist called Nan's name and led her down a carpeted hallway to Dr. Mazzarella's office. He was standing in the doorway to greet her. "Please come in," he said. "I am very glad to meet you."

Dr. Paul Mazzarella was born in Italy, and he received his medical degree in Bologna, but he has been a resident of the United States since he was a teenager. He shares with Dr. Garcia a compassion and sympathy for his patients that inspires their immediate trust. Nan didn't know it but Dr. Mazzarella had some knowledge of the in vitro fertilization procedure when she came to him. Obstetricians and gynecologists in the Manhasset area associated with North Shore University Hospital had been discussing the possibility of setting up an in vitro program. These discussions eventually led to the opening of the in vitro clinic at North Shore University Hospital in January 1983. North Shore's clinic, however, is not a full time in vitro operation. It has had quite a small number of patients compared to the Norfolk program.

Nan sat across the desk from Dr. Mazzarella and was ready to begin with her list of questions when Dr. Mazzarella began asking her questions. "So, tell me," he said. "This is so exciting. What happened?" And he listened without interrupting while Nan told him everything that had happened in Norfolk. At the end, he said, "I can see you have been through a lot." "Yes," said Nan. "As you can see," she continued, "I don't accept the status quo, and I don't take 'no' for an answer. I got this far with this philosophy and I'm not going to change it now when it matters most. I want the absolute best medical care I can buy. If I have to go an hour to New York City every week to get it, I will. Can you give me what I want?"

Dr. Mazzarella studied Nan for a moment; then he said, "If you decide you want us to be your obstetricians, I recommend we be very aggressive about your pregnancy. I don't want you to work, I don't want you to lift anything, no grocery shopping. I want you to rest. You have a normal pregnancy, there should be no complications, but I will follow you very regularly. I will see you every week for the first eighteen weeks, and then we'll reevaluate the situation. I'll call Norfolk for their instructions as soon as you make a decision."

"Those were exactly the words I was looking for," says Nan. "I wanted my obstetrician to approach my pregnancy *aggressively;* he said it." There was no doubt now in Nan's mind. Paul Mazzarella would be her obstetrician. She had to call Dr. Schachter and cancel her appointment.

Nan realized she was afraid to call Dr. Schachter. "I felt disloyal; she'd helped us, and here I was turning her down for another obstetrician. But I really didn't feel comfortable with her." Todd made the call, to cancel the appointment, but that wasn't the end of it. Dr. Schachter called Nan to find out why. "Dr. Jones wants me to be in a high-risk group practice," explained Nan. "I have a group practice," said Dr. Schachter. "I've already made other arrangements," said Nan. "You can't," said Dr. Schachter. "You're my patient." This is what Nan had been afraid of, getting into an argument with her. "I'm sorry," said Nan, hoping to end the discussion. "I'm very grateful for everything you've done for us, but I'm going on the orders of Dr. Jones."

Still, Dr. Schachter persisted. Nan had to tell her. "I just didn't feel comfortable the last time I was in your office. I want a doctor I can feel comfortable with." Then Dr. Schachter asked Nan who she had chosen as her obstetrician. When Nan told her, she hung up. "I felt bad about hurting her," says Nan, "but I wanted the best medical care I could get. I was on the rampage for this baby inside me. I was like a lioness protecting her cubs. You can't make life perfect, but I wanted this situation to be as perfect as I could make it. And that meant having Dr. Mazzarella."

Dr. Mazzarella started seeing Nan Tilton during the first week of August on a regular basis. Dr. Howard Jones did not give Dr. Mazzarella any particular regimen to follow during the pregnancy, except that he continue the Delalutin shots.

Nan had doubts about the Delalutin injections. "I began to be concerned that the progesterone might be having a harmful effect on the embryos, but I trusted the Joneses to know what was best. I prayed it wasn't doing any damage."

Dr. Howard Jones, Jr., also requested that Dr. Mazzarella send blood samples to Norfolk once a month for five months for research purposes. The EVMS was conducting quantitative studies of the pregnancy hormone, human chorionic gonadotropin (HCG). Dr. Jones's last requirement was that an ultrasound examination be made at eight to ten weeks to confirm that the pregnancy was proceeding normally, and the results of this examination were to be sent to Norfolk.

Dr. Mazzarella's approach to Nan's pregnancy differed from his approach to his other patients with normal pregnancies only in that he saw her on a weekly basis. Usually he saw only high-risk patients this frequently. There had been no instructions from Norfolk to treat Nan's pregnancy as a high-risk pregnancy. The decision was Dr. Mazzarella's. "There was nothing wrong medically with Nan's pregnancy," says Dr. Mazzarella. "Once the implantation occurred correctly, Nan's pregnancy could be treated as a normal pregnancy. But we elected to treat it as a high-risk pregnancy due to the modality by which she had gotten pregnant, and for no other reason."

This point of view suited Nan perfectly. She felt the weekly visits to Dr. Mazzarella in the first trimester of her pregnancy would ensure the welfare of the embryos as much as was humanly possible. "The first three months of any pregnancy are crucial," says Dr. Mazzarella. "After three months the likelihood of miscarrying is greatly reduced." The possibility of miscarrying with in vitro fertilization is the same as it is with a pregnancy achieved under normal circumstances.

As for diet, Dr. Mazzarella suggested Nan follow what is considered to be a nutritious diet for anyone—grains, carbohydrates, fruits and vegetables, and low-fat proteins such as chicken and veal. "I asked Nan to avoid sugars because they settle down very quickly as fat," says Dr. Mazzarella. He posed no ceiling on weight gain for pregnancy, but he is concerned that his patients do not gain more than they can easily take off after the baby is born. "The ideal weight gain is about twenty-two pounds," he says.

The cost for Dr. Mazzarella's prenatal care and delivery was $1,500 in 1982. This was his standard price. He did not charge the Tiltons any more because he saw Nan once a week. Todd's insurance covered 80 percent of the costs.

Once Nan knew that she was in competent medical hands, she could concentrate on her role in the pregnancy. She would take care of herself, eat well, stay physically and psychologically healthy, and educate herself so that she'd know enough to be able to detect the first signs of changes or problems, should they arise.

About two weeks after Nan got home from Norfolk, Andrea Nelson called Nan to tell her that she had lost her baby. She miscarried four weeks after the transfer. "She was hysterical, out of her mind," says Nan. "She looked for everything she could find to blame it on." Nan felt Andrea had lost the baby because she didn't take it easy when she got home from Norfolk. Nan had done little else herself but go to the doctor since she'd come home. The rest of the time she had spent lying down. Todd was doing the grocery shopping. They'd been eating sandwiches for dinner so Nan wouldn't have to cook. Andrea Nelson's misfortune only reinforced Nan's resolve to spend as much of the next nine months in bed as possible.

Following Dr. Mazzarella's orders not to work, Nan wrote a letter of resignation to Friends Academy. "The principal was happy for me, but it was August, only a month before school started. It was a little late to be telling him I wasn't going to be teaching that year."

On August 11, four weeks after Nan's embryo transfer, she went for her weekly visit to Dr. Mazzarella and for the first time heard through a Doppler, an ultrasonic instrument, the sound of blood flowing through the uterus to the developing embryos. Nan went for her next visit on August 18. Everything was proceeding normally, Dr. Mazzarella assured her.

That night, Nan was putting on her nightgown when she saw a bloody brown discharge in her underpants. "Todd," she shrieked. He came running up the stairs. Together they looked at the spot. Nan didn't want to call the doctor until she knew what was happening. She got out all of her pregnancy books to see what they had to say. Bleeding is not unusual in pregnant women, they discovered. Twenty percent of pregnant women have some bleeding and it can occur around the time of their menstrual period. "Todd and I got into bed," says Nan, "and held onto each other for dear life."

In the morning when Nan woke up, she still had a bloody brown discharge. She called Dr. Mazzarella right away. By the time he called her back, the bleeding had stopped. Dr. Mazzarella told her it was nothing to worry about unless it continued or the discharge became more abundant; then she was to call him immediately.

On Monday, August 23, Nan sent her monthly blood sample to Norfolk. Dr. Mazzarella decided to do Nan's first ultrasound that week. He arranged an appointment for her the next day. Tuesday, August 24, Todd stayed home from work to go with Nan to the hospital for the exam. The purpose of an ultrasound exam during pregnancy is to determine how well the fetus is developing. With ultrasound, doctors can measure the head size, the abdominal size, and the length of the femur bone in the leg of the fetus, and compare those measurements with the measurements that have been established as the norm for that stage of gestational development. A normal pregnancy does not require an ultrasound examination, but obstetricians are using them more routinely now that the technology is available to establish with greater certainty the gestational age of the fetus. If for any reason an obstetrician suspects that the fetus is not developing on schedule, an ultrasound can provide information that will be helpful in confirming or negating this suspicion.

Nan was an old hand at ultrasound exams by now. She had started drinking water before she left for the hospital where the exam was to be done. She even took a jug of water along with her in the car. "I wanted to be full, just right when I got there so I didn't have to wait for the exam and have all that pressure on my bladder."

Dr. Mazzarella was waiting for them in the hallway when they arrived. He met Todd for the first time and then introduced the Tiltons to Dr. Mitchell Goldman, head of the Ultrasound Department. "All the top guys in the hospital were there to see this ultrasound," says Todd. Nan went into the examining room. They were going to bring in Todd when everything was set. Dr. Mazzarella held Nan's hand while Dr. Goldman was adjusting the ultrasound equipment. Goldman was completing his preparations when he commented casually, "Well, I see two already, an instant family." Nan thought she hadn't understood. "Two?" she asked. "Two what?" "Two babies," said Dr. Mazzarella. "Twins." "It's twins?" squealed Nan. "Oh, my God, I can't believe it. Where's Todd? Get Todd in here."

Todd came in the door and the first thing he heard was "twins." "It's twins?" he said. *"Two babies,"* cried Nan. *"Two babies."* "My God," said Todd. Dr. Goldman pointed to two little sacs on the screen that contained the embryos. It was hard to make them out. Ultrasound images are grainy black and white. But then Todd saw them, two little hearts beating. "They looked like moth wings flickering on the screen."

"What's that?" asked Todd, pointing to another dark spot on the screen. "We suspect that it is a third embryo which began to grow but did not survive," said Dr. Goldman. "She might have miscarried that third embryo when she had the bleeding," said Dr. Mazzarella. Nan never saw that little spot on the ultrasound screen, fortunately. But Todd had and it haunted him for weeks afterward. "I kept thinking about the baby we'd lost," says Todd.

Nan could only think about the two babies growing inside her. "All we'd ever wanted, Todd and I, was a baby of our own. Now we were going to have *two*. It seemed almost like too much. To be the beneficiaries of such good fortune was overwhelming."

As soon as Nan and Todd got home from the hospital, they called Dr. Garcia in Norfolk to tell him the news. "I'll never forget what he said," says Nan. "He said, 'It's too early to get excited about twins.' 'But I saw them on the screen,' I said. 'Your first trimester isn't over yet,' he said. 'We don't know what will happen.' "

Nan hung up the telephone and she was furious. "I was so happy," she says. "I wanted to fly. It wasn't the time to be realistic. I wanted him to be happy too." Nan found out later that as usual, Dr. Garcia had his reasons. He had told another patient she was having twins and then she lost one in the first trimester. Nan had four more weeks to go before she would complete her first trimester.

Nan Tilton had three more ultrasounds during her pregnancy. Each time, the head sizes of the babies were right on the mark, right where they should be for that stage of the babies' development. "Although we can't be certain," Dr. Mazzarella told Nan, "this is an indication that you will have fine, healthy babies." The ultrasound also confirmed Nan's due date: April 5.

When the ultrasound revealed that Nan was carrying twins, Dr. Mazzarella put Nan on a regimen of increasing bed rest, beginning in the middle of her fifth month. By the end of the nine months, Nan was resting almost all the time, except for her visits to Dr. Mazzarella. "It's the technique that the old-fashioned obstetricians used to use," says Dr. Mazzarella. "I'm still convinced that it's the best way to treat multiple gestations. When we treat multiple pregnancies with bed rest, they are more likely to come to term."

While obligatory bed rest for four months might have been a hardship for someone as active as Nan Tilton in other circumstances, she never uttered a word of complaint. "You ask a woman who wants a child badly to do anything and she'll do it," says Dr. Mazzarella. Once Nan had chosen Dr. Mazzarella as her obstetrician, she never questioned anything he did. "I trusted him the way I trusted Dr. Garcia," says Nan. "He was going to make it work." Nan went home from his office each week secure in the knowledge she was being well cared for and the babies were progressing as they should.

At home Nan did her part. She rested and she ate. She followed Dr. Mazzarella's instructions about diet and supplemented his diet with the diet prescribed in the book *Having Twins* by Elizabeth Noble, published by Houghton Mifflin in 1980. It is a comprehensive guide to prenatal and postnatal care for expectant mothers of twins. For the first three months, Nan felt nauseated every afternoon around four. "It was like getting the flu." The nausea usually went away about eleven at night, then Nan was hungry. After three months, the nausea subsided and Nan felt well all day long. She ate three big meals a day, a snack in the afternoon, a protein drink made out of milk and bananas before she went to bed at eleven, and she often got up in the middle of the night for a snack. "I was hungry," says Nan. "I couldn't make it through the night without eating."

Nan was convinced she could increase the babies' birth weight by eating. "I was nurturing those babies inside me," says Nan. "I was determined they were going to be at least six pounds at birth. I didn't want it to look like there was something wrong with the in vitro process. If they weighed under five pounds and they had to be put into an incubator when they were born, everyone would blame it on the in vitro technique."

"I told Nan many times, there is no connection between the amount of weight the pregnant mother gains and the birth weight of her baby," says Dr. Mazzarella. "Birth weight is determined primarily by genetics. Low birth weights have been shown to result when the mother smokes or drinks on a regular basis; it has nothing to do with the mother's diet."

Nan did not listen to him. By the end of her first three months, Nan had gained fifteen pounds. "I was wearing maternity clothes in September," says Nan. This was already about 75 percent of the weight most women gain in nine months. Every week in Dr. Mazzarella's office, the nurse weighed Nan. "She'd say, 'Dr. Mazzarella is going to kill you,' but he never even mentioned it," says Nan. "I closed both my eyes and both my ears and let Nan do what she wanted," says Dr. Mazzarella. "She was a very motivated woman. I knew she would take off the weight when she had two babies to chase after."

At the end of October, Dr. Mazzarella told Nan she had passed the danger point. It was less likely that she would miscarry now. He didn't need to see her every week. She was to come to his office every two weeks for the next five months. Nan was certain at this point that she would carry the two babies to term. "That's when I started talking to them," says Nan.

Nan was reading all the time, everything she could get her hands on about pregnancy and birth. She'd found a book called *The Secret Life of the Unborn Child*, by Thomas Verny, M.D., and John Kelly, published by Delta Books in 1981. Verny and Kelly say the fetus growing inside the mother is sensitive to the world outside the womb as well as the mother's psychological state. So Nan sat for hours in her bed, rubbing her stomach, caressing the babies inside her. "I'd say, 'Mommy loves you, Mommy loves you,'" says Nan. "It got to be a joke. Everyone laughed because I always had my hands on my stomach."

Nan never minded that people looked at her. "I loved it," says Nan.

"I relished their attention. I showed off, I paraded around. In the grocery store, I was the one who was pregnant now and the other women were looking at me."

In the fourth month of her pregnancy, Nan decided that she didn't want to take the risk of something going wrong during the delivery. She asked Dr. Mazzarella if he would deliver the babies by Caesarian section. Dr. Mazzarella was reluctant to do it unless it was medically indicated. He told Nan he would postpone making a decision until later in her pregnancy. Nan signed up for Lamaze classes on natural childbirth to begin in February.

One Sunday in the fifth month of her pregnancy, Nan went to the Friends Meeting alone. Todd stayed home to do some work for the office. By the strangest chance, there were only women at Meeting that day. It had never happened at Meeting before, nor has it happened since. It is the practice at Friends Meeting to sit quietly. When a Friend has something to share, he or she stands up and offers his or her thoughts to the Meeting.

A woman stood up and commented on the fact of there being only women present, and she related an incident that illustrated the strength and courage of women. Nan was moved to stand up then and tell the story of hers and Todd's infertility. At the end she said, "It was by coming to Meeting, being with you and receiving guidance from God, that I knew I should persevere. The doctors said it was impossible, but I am pregnant now and having twins." She sat down and another member of the Meeting stood up. "On behalf of us here and the members of the Matinecock Meeting, we give you our best wishes for this wonderful news."

When she had finished, Nan heard a man's voice. She turned around and behind her was one lone man who had come in late. "My wife and I too had a difficult time having a child," he said. "We waited eight years before we had our first child. Even though I am a man, I know what the experience of infertility is like. At the time, it seems as though there is nothing else in your life. But now, I look back on those eight years alone with my wife as something special. You'll know what I mean someday. Everything happens in its time."

When Nan got home, she slipped into the house quietly so as not to disturb Todd. She wanted to think about what the man at Meeting had said. She and Todd hardly talked to each other anymore. It was always the babies, the babies. Nan was concentrating so intensely on the future. Were she and Todd losing this last chance to enjoy each other alone?

Maybe women who didn't have infertility problems were more aware of what they were giving up by having a child. Todd had been doing so much for her. She thought it was what he wanted too. Was it?

Nan went upstairs to Todd's office and looked in the door. He was concentrating on what he was doing. He looked up and smiled at her. Nan went over to him and put her hand on the back of his neck, where his muscles knotted when he was tense. She stood behind him, massaging the tension away. "Let's go out to dinner tonight," Nan suggested, knowing he would like to. "Do you really want to?" asked Todd, knowing she was obsessed about staying home. They went out and they were both glad. It reminded them that they enjoyed each other's company. They would do it more often, they agreed. But time was growing short.

Nan dreamed that night that she was out in the backyard with her two little boys. They were begging her to let them ride around the block on their bicycles by themselves. They'd done it many times before, but always with her. She reluctantly agreed to let them do it. Gleefully they got on their bicycles and took off down the street. Nan watched them disappear from sight, then waited for them to come back. She waited and waited, watching, and they never came back.

When Nan was thirty-two weeks pregnant, in her eighth month, Dr. Mazzarella sent Nan to North Shore University Hospital for her fourth ultrasound. It showed that one of the babies was lying in the transverse position, sideways across the uterus instead of head pointing down, and was in breech presentation. The position of the babies made a natural delivery an impossibility.

"I would have to deliver the babies by Caesarian section," says Dr. Mazzarella. He scheduled the birth for March 24, 1983, about two weeks before Nan would have gone into labor.

By the time Nan was in her ninth month, she had gained seventy-two pounds. "When Nan does something," says Todd, "she does it all the way." She could not move easily by herself. Todd pushed her around the house on a chair. Her stomach was so big, she was physically unable to bend over. "I got really good at doing things with me feet," says Nan. "I could work the stereo, the TV with my toes; I could put on my under-pants and get them up to my knees with my toes. I could even pick up a business card on the floor with my toes." Nan couldn't see her feet unless she was lying down. To shave her legs, she taped a razor onto a ruler and did it lying down. "I was so fat I had jowls and a double chin. People who knew me were shocked. I liked it."

The last month Nan and Todd spent getting the babies' room ready. Todd's parents and Nan's parents both helped. They painted the room beige and bought two identical white cribs. Nan had found an antique crib early in her pregnancy; they put that in their bedroom. Deciding on names was a big problem. They had to come up with two names for each sex. Everyone was convinced that the Tiltons would have two boys. "The heartbeats were fast, Nan's shape, all those superstitions," says Todd. They had thought of two boys names—Jeffrey Keith Tilton, and Christopher James Tilton. But they only came up with one girl's name—Heather. "I was convinced," says Todd, "that we were having two of the same sex, but neither one of us ever considered that it might be two girls."

Todd drove Nan to North Shore University Hospital on the afternoon of March 23. "We were really going this time to have a baby," says Nan, remembering the other time when she had gone for her first laparoscopy. Everyone on the hospital staff seemed to know who the Tiltons were, and every one of them found an excuse to go into Nan's room that night.

At nine o'clock, Dr. Mazzarella came in. Nan wanted to be sure that Todd was going to be given special permission to be in the operating room for the delivery. The hospital's policy was not to let husbands into the operating room for Caesarian sections. "I'm working on it," Dr. Mazzarella assured her. Nan was surprised. She thought everything had been settled.

At nine-thirty, Nan was finally alone. She thought how different everything would be the next day. She would know all the things any mother knows when her babies have been delivered. She would know if they were healthy; she would know what sex they were; and she'd know what they looked like. She wrote a letter to her unborn children that night.

I am writing this on March 23, 1983, the night before you are to be born. It is 9:30. I am in the hospital. Daddy has just gone home and we have shared the whole day together, thinking about how lucky we are to have you both coming. Our doctors from Norfolk called us today and wished us well and wanted us to know again what a miracle you are. Daddy and I know that God wanted us to have you and he gave us the strength and the courage we needed to find a way to do it. Daddy and I wish you a Happy Birthday and look forward to holding you in our arms for the very first time and beginning our new lives together with you.

Nan was awake by five the next morning. She got up and went down the hall to take a shower. The nurses and the hospital doctors kept coming in to check Nan's temperature and her blood pressure, and they hooked her up to a fetal monitor. At seven-fifteen, Dr. Mazzarella came by her room and told her he'd be back at ten to deliver the babies. "Everything's all set for Todd," he said. Todd arrived at eight-thirty.

An hour later, the nurse came with a wheelchair to take her to the operating room. Todd walked along beside her, holding her hand. At the door of the operating room, the nurse said, "Okay, Mrs. Tilton, kiss your husband good-bye; he'll wait here." "Wait a minute," said Nan. "That's not the plan." "We have special permission," said Todd. "That's absolutely impossible," said the nurse. "We never allow husbands to be present for Caesarian births," and she left them outside the door while she went in search of a doctor. Just then Michael Gilbert, the Tiltons' pediatrician, arrived. His presence was required at the birth to examine the babies as soon as they were born. He had brought with him two pediatricians from the hospital's department of neonatology to be standing by in case they were needed.

The nurse came back then and said she was waiting to get approval from the Chief of Surgery before she admitted Todd to the operating room. "At this point," says Todd, "I didn't want to make a big issue about it. I really wanted to be with Nan, but I didn't want to rock the boat so that it would create a problem for anyone on the hospital staff."

It was Nan who did the fighting. "We'd been through so much together," she says. "For him to miss out on this part was unbearable to me. I wanted Todd to be there to start the connection with our children, to hold them and have that bonding take place."

Todd stayed outside the operating room. The nurse wheeled Nan inside and she got up on the table. The incision for a Caesarian section is made right along the pubic hairline. On Nan it would be very close to the scar that remained from her laparotomy in Norfolk. The scar was long and it had healed in a ridge. Dr. Mazzarella told Nan that he would fix the scar during the Caesarian surgery.

The nurse prepared Nan for the surgery by shaving the pubic hair an inch down from the hairline; then the anesthesiologist came in. He would be giving Nan an epidural anesthesia. It would numb the lower part of her body. Nan would be awake during the operation, but would not feel anything. The anesthesiologist asked Nan to lie on her side and curl up in a ball. "I was so huge," says Nan, "they didn't think I'd be able to do it. The nurses said they'd never seen anyone so big." This time Nan felt none of the nervousness she'd felt during her other operations. "I was so excited. It was like waiting at the airport for someone to come. I wanted to *see* those babies, to hold them in my arms."

Dr. Mazzarella came in then, singing, "Oh, what a beautiful morning . . ." With him was his associate, Dr. Howard Kraft. Dr. Mazzarella put his hands on Nan's stomach. "At least six pounds each," he said. Then the nurses put up a screen, right under Nan's chin so that she could not see what the doctors were doing. At the very last minute, just before Dr. Mazzarella made the incision, word came down from the Hospital Board that Todd Tilton was permitted in the operating room. The nurses helped him get into a sterile gown and mask, and hurried him into the room. He came around to stand by Nan's head and hold her hand. "He looked so funny wearing one of those surgical shower caps," says Nan.

Todd tried to distract Nan by talking about sailing. Then Nan felt something. "It hurts," she said. "Let's breathe," said Todd and he guided her in the Lamaze breathing technique they had learned at the first Lamaze class. The anesthesiologist was concerned. He pricked her toes with a pin. "Can you feel that?" he asked. She could. "I guess I'll have to give you some more," he said. Nan could feel the anesthesia going into her back and told him. "You must be very sensitive," he said. "It felt like someone was wrenching my pubic bone," says Nan.

While the doctors were working, the nurse was giving Nan a blow-by-blow description of what they were doing. "They're moving the liver now," she said. Nan told her to spare the gory details. "They can see the babies now," the nurse said, "They can see one of the babies . . . one of the babies is about to be born . . . one baby is about to be born . . . You have a little girl."

"Oh, my God," said Nan and Todd at the same time, crying. "I never thought I'd have a *little girl,*" said Nan. "That was so much more than we'd expected, a little girl." And then Nan heard the baby crying. It was at that moment that Nan finally believed that she was having a baby. "A little girl," wept Nan, "somebody to make cookies with at Christmas." It was ten fifty-seven. The pediatrician took the baby immediately to the other side of the room, where they checked her color, respiration, heart rate, reflexes, and muscular response. "I can see her," said Todd. "She's beautiful."

Sixty seconds later the nurse announced, "You have a little boy." Nan noticed immediately that his cry was different. And then Nan was out. The doctor had put her under general anesthesia to do the stitching. She didn't know anything else; she still hadn't even seen the babies when she woke up an hour later in the recovery room.

Todd, though, saw what happened next. The girl was lying on one table with a pediatrician standing over her, and the boy was lying on another table. The doctor examining the girl made a sign to indicate that she was all right, then all of the pediatricians in the delivery room went over to the boy. "It looked as if they thought something was wrong with him," says Todd. He went over to the doctors to find out what was happening when nurses whisked both babies away to the nursery. Todd followed the nurses down the hall. He stood outside the nursery and watched through the window while a nurse gave Todd Jr. his first bath. "It was fantastic," says Todd. "I saw the whole thing; she did it right there in front of me. The baby looked all right to me but what did I know?"

Todd waited until the pediatrician came out of the nursery to ask if there was something wrong. The pediatrician muttered something about not being satisfied with the way the male baby was responding. "I was really worried then," says Todd. "I went into the recovery room to wait for Nan to come out of the anesthesia and I prayed. When Nan woke up, I told her."

"Is he retarded?" Nan screamed. Dr. Mazzarella heard her and came into the room. "What's the matter?" he asked. "Is he retarded?" yelled Nan again. Dr. Mazzarella rushed out the door to the nursery. He was back again a few minutes later. "Everything is fine," he assured Nan. "The pediatrician wasn't pleased with his color at first, but he's responding very well now."

Nan did not see her babies until two o'clock that afternoon. Dr. Mazzarella came to Recovery and personally wheeled Nan down to the nursery. Two nurses stood in the doorway, waiting for Nan; each one of them was holding a baby. A nurse put Todd Jr. in Nan's arms first. "I looked down at that adorable little face," says Nan, "and it was the face I'd seen in my dreams." She held Todd to her cheek. "I've waited so long for you," Nan whispered. "Mommy loves you so much." She stayed like that without moving, murmuring to Todd until the nurse put Heather into her arms. Nan was astounded. "This baby was a child from heaven," says Nan. "She didn't look like anyone we knew. She had dark, almost jet black hair and a round cherubic face with bright pink cheeks. I could never even have dreamed such a face."

Nan knew instinctively exactly what to do. She put the babies to her breasts, one on each side, and they nursed right away. The tears ran sideways down Nan's cheeks into her ears.

Heather and Todd Tilton were the eighteenth and nineteenth children to be conceived and born by in vitro fertilization at the Eastern Virginia Medical School's VIP Program, and the first in vitro twins born in the United States. They each weighed seven pounds.

The Tiltons kept the press away for four days. On March 28, they held a press conference in the auditorium of North Shore University Hospital. The pediatrician, Michael Gilbert, demanded that the press be kept at least twenty feet away from the babies. There was a rope strung across the room to ensure that the press complied with this condition. The twins were brought into the auditorium in small covered cribs called isolettes. Nan and Todd each held one baby briefly for photographs, then the babies were taken back to the nursery. Nan and Todd wanted to be certain that there was no confusion in the minds of the press that it was the Eastern Virginia Medical School in vitro program that was responsible for the births, not North Shore Hospital. Therefore Dr. Jairo Garcia had flown up from Norfolk to be present at the press conference and answer questions about the in vitro procedure. It was then that Nan and Todd learned how really fortunate they were. "The Tiltons are very lucky," Dr. Garcia told the press. "There is only an 8 percent chance of carrying two babies to term, even with four embryos transferred." Now Nan knew why up until the very end Dr. Garcia had been so discouraging. She blessed him for it, for not telling her.

The next day the headlines hit the national newspapers. "Test-Tube Twins Born." From that moment, there was a constant stream of people passing by the nursery and Nan's room—hospital staff, other patients, visitors. That night the twins were moved to a separate nursery where they were no longer on public view. Security guards were put outside Nan's room and the twins' nursery.

Nan and Todd Tilton took Heather and Todd home from the hospital on March 30, 1983. "Finally the babies were in our control," says Nan. "We'd had to rely on doctors to do everything for us until then. Now they were *our* babies, our very own babies."

After all the relatives and friends had been notified, after the press had had its turn, the last person Todd Tilton called to tell about the twins was his high school biology teacher. She was surprised to hear from him.

She hadn't had any contact with him since he had graduated fifteen years before. "It was *you*," Todd told her, "you who taught me so well about human reproduction. When I found out what in vitro fertilization was, it made sense. I knew it was right for Nan and me. Thank you."

One Year Later

On March 24, 1984, Heather and Todd Tilton were one year old. The press started calling the month before to set up photo sessions with America's first test-tube twins. The public is interested in them because they represent a significant advance in medical science—in vitro fertilization.

Their parents, however, tend to forget that. They are Heather and Todd, their children. Heather is as dark as Todd is fair. Nan and Todd Tilton's efforts now are concentrated on bringing up their children, and coping with the conflicts between husband and wife that inevitably accompany the adjustments that must be made during the first years of a child's life. *"He* doesn't spend enough time with the kids," she says. *"She* doesn't spend enough time with me," he says.

In May 1984, when the twins were fourteen months old, Nan and Todd took the twins to Norfolk for a thorough physical evaluation. It is not an obligatory visit; the purpose was to gather data needed to establish that in vitro fertilization produces healthy, normal children. As of May 1984, the Children's Hospital of The King's Daughters in Norfolk had evaluated sixteen in vitro children. "We will have to see more than two hundred before we can be sure there are no genetic risks in in vitro fertilization," says Dr. Frederick Wirth, Director of Neonatology at Children's Hospital. Children's Hospital in Norfolk is the only hospital in the world evaluating in vitro children.

The second and no less important reason for the evaluation was to reassure the parents of in vitro children that their babies are healthy and normal in all stages of development. The cost for this evaluation in May 1984 was $477.46. About half of that amount was paid by the Tiltons' insurance. The rest was paid by the hospital. The participating doctors charged no professional fees for their work.

The Tiltons never hesitated a moment to cooperate with the EVMS VIP Program in this endeavor. "What the Joneses and Dr. Garcia had done for us we could never repay," says Nan Tilton. "We wanted to do something for them. If we could help substantiate the efficacy and the success of in vitro fertilization, we would do it. We have the living proof that it works."

Pediatricians at the hospital had arranged a two-day barrage of tests for the twins, beginning with a general checkup to assess their overall health, then a neurological examination, to be followed by a psychological developmental evaluation in the afternoon. The following day, the twins would be given ultrasound examinations of the heart and lungs, brain and abdomen. At the end of the two-day evaluation, there would be a press conference.

Nan Tilton remembers vividly walking through the Norfolk airport that May morning. With her she had two strollers, two diaper bags, and two toddlers—Heather insisting on walking, Todd determined to have his bottle. She would never forget how she had felt the last time she had been in the Norfolk airport. "I sat alone right there in that coffee shop," said Nan, pointing with her elbow, "waiting for my flight back to New York, thinking nobody knows what I have growing inside me right now. The embryos were then nine days old. I didn't know them. I know them now, and they're not even babies anymore."

It was twelve o'clock when Nan and Todd drove up in triumph to the front of the Omni Hotel in their rented station wagon with its two rented car seats. There was no one to notice that they had come back with children this time. Their very anonymity was the icing on the cake. "See," says Nan. "We were normal now. We had kids. No one even looked at us."

The lounge and piano bar where Nan had spent so much time was still there, but the coffee shop and bar were gone. There was a new outdoor café overlooking the harbor, and next to the hotel was a brand-new Waterside complex of restaurants, boutiques, and fast food places. "This must be where the girls spend their time now," said Nan, looking around for them. But the VIP Program was between sessions. Session 15 would begin at the end of the week.

Over at Medical Tower, however, there were people waiting to welcome the Tiltons: Linda Lynch, Doris, Dr. Garcia, Dr. Howard Jones, Jr., Dr. Georgeanna Jones, all crowded into the new waiting room where, beginning with the next series of patients, the nurses would draw the daily blood samples.

"We have 106 patients coming in our next series, all within five weeks," Dr. Howard Jones, Jr. told Nan. "We've got to have someplace to put them." While Nan was at Norfolk, the VIP Program had treated 60 patients in a seven-week period. "We've increased our enrollment 35 percent and added one doctor," Dr. Jones said.

Nan could see that the heavier workload was taking its toll. Dr. Garcia seemed to have aged considerably in a year. "He looked so tired," says Nan. "He didn't have that gray forelock before."

"We are extremely overloaded with work," says Dr. Garcia. "We start before seven in the morning and we go until late in the evening. We work holidays, weekends; we feel physically tired. We feel the burden of working at that pace. And because I see the patients every day, I get involved in their emotional and economic problems. But when I see the Tiltons' faces, I know it has been worthwhile."

The entire VIP in vitro team took turns holding Heather and Todd. Linda Lynch had just gotten a new camera, so she recorded the twins' homecoming on film. There were a few tears and many smiles as the assembled company silently celebrated the miracle in which they had participated.

For the next two days, Heather and Todd Tilton, while accorded all the pomp and ceremony of visiting dignitaries, were ignobly undressed and dressed, poked and pulled, squirted with mineral oil, and charged with tasks such as putting nine red cubes into a cup. Through it all they remained marvelously good-humored, generous with their smiles, and eager to greet each new doctor. Nan and Todd were the epitome of grace under pressure. While any other parents might have called a halt to the proceedings after the third examination, Nan and Todd gritted their teeth and demonstrated the same easygoing personalities as their children.

Only at the end, in front of the television cameras and international press, did the children collapse, and no amount of balloons, life-sized stuffed bears, or parental entreaties could coax them out of it. They had had it. Unlike the twins, Nan and Todd looked like a storybook American couple: feeling blessed, they rose to the occasion. In a few words, they articulated the anguish, solitude, and suffering of an infertile couple, and celebrated the miracle they had been given.

The doctors who had examined Heather and Todd Tilton pronounced the children to be physically and psychologically sound: Dr. Frederick Wirth, Dr. L. Matthew Frank, pediatric neurologist, Dr. Rufus Jennings, pediatric cardiologist, Dr. Harry Presberg, pediatric radiologist, and Virginia Van de Water, school psychologist.

"We found no birth or genetic defects," said spokesman Wirth.

"They are within the normal range of physical development, having met all developmental milestones. Their personalities were found to be moderate to easygoing, coordinated in relating to other people. In mental development, they are above average; both tested at the nineteen-month-old level. In motor development, Todd is slightly more advanced than Heather. He tested at the level of sixteen months old, Heather at fifteen months. They are off to a very good start."

Dr. Jairo Garcia and Drs. Howard and Georgeanna Jones had known the twins would come through the evaluation with flying colors. "We haven't had a single in vitro child with genetic or birth defects," says Dr. Howard Jones, Jr. "In fact, we find that our in vitro babies rate very high on the developmental scale. It is an indication that the patients we treat are above average in intelligence." It is also an indication of the biggest limitation of the in vitro procedure as it is practiced in this country—it is restricted to only those couples who can afford its high cost. Until insurance companies are willing to remove the in vitro procedure from the realm of experimental procedures and acknowledge it as valid medical practice, in vitro fertilization will be available only to the affluent. "Artificial insemination is covered almost 90 percent by insurance," says Dr. Howard Jones, Jr. "Why can't the major insurance companies cover in vitro?"

When the camera lights were turned off, and the Tiltons were in the privacy of their hotel room, Nan felt great relief. In spite of everything she and Todd had been through in the years of their infertility, and the in vitro process itself, Nan tended to forget how the children had been conceived. "When we're at home," says Nan, "Heather and Todd are just our children. Down in Norfolk, they seemed like freaks, a product of medical science, not a product of our bodies. Today they are miracle babies. But by the time they grow up, there will be thousands of in vitro children, and the fact that they were conceived in a petri dish will not even be worth mentioning."

That time, however, is still far off. By April 30, 1984, the official count, as reported at the Third International Conference on In Vitro Fertilization in Helsinki, was 512 births and 588 babies born by in vitro fertilization around the world. The majority of them have been conceived at four in vitro programs—the Eastern Virginia Medical School's VIP Program, Steptoe and Edwards' clinic at Bourne Hall in Cambridge, England, and the two Australian groups in Melbourne, Monash University and the University of Melbourne. There were 56 sets of twins, 7 sets of triplets, and 2 sets of quadruplets.

By that same date, the EVMS VIP Program, since renamed The Howard and Georgeanna Jones Institute for Reproductive Medicine, had produced 54 babies in 52 births. At the end of 1984, the VIP Program had treated 509 patients since its inception in 1980 and performed 900 or so egg retrievals. In May 1985, the Institute celebrated its 117th birth. Based on the number of embryos transferred, the pregnancy rate at Norfolk is currently 26.3 percent.

The statistics of overall success for the program's operation don't tell the real story of the clinic's success. "In a recent cycle," says Dr. Garcia, "we had a 46 percent pregnancy rate. This is astonishing when you remember we finished our first year with a pregnancy rate of 13 percent."

Another factor which influences the pregnancy rate is that each group of patients is made up of patients with very different infertility problems. For example, the male factor group—couples with low sperm counts—have a much lower chance of getting pregnant than couples with other kinds of infertility problems. "In our male factor group, there is something in the patient's sperm that prevents them from penetrating the egg and fertilizing it. We've had fertilization in about half our patients with low sperm counts," says Dr. Garcia. "We might come up with the right *amount* of sperm, but we need *quality* sperm. In Mr. Tilton's case, he had a high enough sperm count to come up with enough quality sperm to fertilize the eggs." Still, the quantity of sperm required is much less than it would be in normal fertilization. "We've had eggs fertilize routinely with sperm concentrations of 50,000 per milliliter," says Dr. Howard Jones, Jr., "and we've gotten fertilization with 12,500, but none lower."

In other patient groups, the pregnancy rate is much higher. "Our highest pregnancy rates," says Dr. Garcia, "are among patients who have endometriosis, a patient group we began accepting in 1983, and among those patients whom we classify as 'normal infertile.' For our normal infertile group, our pregnancy rate is 34 percent. Our endometriosis patients have a 29.2 percent pregnancy rate. The chances of pregnancy are also very high among patients in the male factor group *if* the husband's sperm fertilizes the egg. Nan and Todd Tilton were in this group. The pregnancy rate for this group is 21.8 percent, based on the number of embryos transferred."

The pregnancy rate also improves from year to year. In the first year, the VIP Program's success rate was 13.2 percent. In 1982, the pregnancy rate was 16.5 percent. In 1983, it was 21.3 percent, and by the end of 1984, it was 23.4 percent, per egg retrieval.

On any given cycle of patients, however, the chances of pregnancy being achieved are related to the number of eggs recruited and embryos that are transferred. "We know very well," says Dr. Garcia, "that when only one embryo is transferred, the chances are about 20 percent that the patient will become pregnant. If we transfer three embryos, our chances are 38 percent; with four embryos, it's close to 40 percent. If we transfer six or more embryos, our chances are as high as 50 percent that pregnancy will occur." Therefore, it is clear that the more follicles the ovary can be stimulated to produce, the higher the chances are that pregnancy will be achieved. "It's simple," says Dr. Howard Jones, Jr. "The success of in vitro fertilization depends on consistently being able to transfer multiple embryos."

What all these statistics mean to the individual in vitro patient is that the process of in vitro fertilization is a process of "keep trying." "This is the story of human reproduction," explains Dr. Garcia. "Through the in vitro process, we see the same statistical curve for pregnancy rates as we see in the process of natural intercourse, but with one big difference. Normal, fertile couples who try every month—90 percent of them will be pregnant by the end of the first year. Through in vitro fertilization, 90 percent of our patients are pregnant within six months of trying; 30 percent of our pregnancies occur in the first in vitro attempt, 50 percent after three trials, and 90 percent after six trials."

The success rate of The Howard and Georgeanna Jones Institute parallels the pregnancy rate of Steptoe and Edwards in England. Steptoe and Edwards are now using the hormone stimulated method too. Various programs around the world are beginning to report similar success rates, using a technique similar to the Joneses' method. But in the United States, the Norfolk program is unique. According to The American Fertility Society, there are now about eighty-five in vitro fertilization programs in this country alone, and not one of them has approached the success of the Jones Institute. Many have still to achieve their first pregnancy.

Howard and Georgeanna Jones feel that the success of their program is due to the individualized treatment that each patient receives. "There is no way an in vitro program can give every patient the same treatment and get the results we're getting," says Dr. Howard Jones, Jr. "We can't emphasize this enough. Every patient has a different response to the hormone stimulation. If you administer the same doses of the same hormone to every patient, you are going to lose 25 to 30 percent of your patients because they won't respond. When we fit the treatment to each patient, we seem to be giving the greatest chance of getting pregnant to the greatest number of our patients."

But in addition to the individualized clinical approach to their patients, the Norfolk in vitro team also has a personal involvement with each one of its patients. "We try to keep our program as warm and as personal as possible," says Dr. Garcia. "Every patient counts. Every patient has a special place in our program and with each of the doctors. This kind of approach makes the work difficult, but that's why, I believe, we have been successful."

It is the Joneses who have established this humanistic approach to in vitro fertilization in Norfolk. "Dr. Howard Jones brought together a group of people for his in vitro team who had principles, who had values," explains Dr. Garcia. "These are not to be found in the medical books. They are things one acquires early in life. In my country, Colombia, the humanistic values are more important than anything else. Here I have found others who believe the same thing."

Dr. Howard Jones, Jr., and Dr. Georgeanna Jones feel very strongly that what they've learned about making in vitro fertilization work should be shared with other in vitro programs around the world. For this reason, they hold monthly seminars in Norfolk for medical professionals and administrators, to explain their approach and their technique. Visitors are invited into the operating room to see an egg retrieval, and they may watch the egg retrieval and transfer procedures as they are being done, on closed circuit television. Visitors are given a tour of the embryology laboratory, the andrology and endocrinology labs, the computer facility, and they go home with a catalogue of every piece of equipment used in the operating room and laboratories by brand name and order number, copies of the blank record sheets used to record data on each patient from hormone treatment to transfer, and research papers on the latest findings in the areas of research in which the institute is engaged.

While other in vitro programs are quick to go out and buy the itemized equipment, many are unwilling to adopt the fundamental element of Norfolk's success—the twenty-four-hour-a-day monitoring and treatment of each individual patient, weekends, holidays, all year round. Other reasons which might explain the lack of success at other in vitro clinics is that they are less well known, and they don't get the volume of patients that the Joneses get. Therefore their pregnancy rate is bound to be lower. "We don't get enough patients to be able to predict reliably how they will respond to the hormone stimulation," says the director of a Southern university's in vitro facility. "We also have a high percentage of subop-timal patients. Their average age is higher and their infertility problems are more complex. They are the hard-to-treat cases."

"We put a lot more emphasis on ultrasound," says a spokesman for an in vitro program in New England. "We depend on ultrasound almost entirely to determine when a patient is ready for egg retrieval. We gave up looking at the cervical mucus. It's too much of a nuisance. We draw blood, do ultrasounds, but no pelvic exams. I think we do need to individualize our program, but that makes it expensive."

Based on their five years of experience with in vitro fertilization, the Joneses and the staff at the Institute for Reproductive Medicine are con-tinually modifying their techniques. Their goal is to get as many eggs as possible for retrieval and fertilization. With patients who over a period of three or four in vitro attempts have failed continually to respond to the hormone stimulation in the Pergonal-FSH combination, Dr. Georgeanna Jones began in July 1983 to administer pure FSH alone. "It means these patients are not getting any luteinizing hormone at all," says Dr. George-anna Jones, "which is what Pergonal contains along with FSH. We get just as high estrogen levels without it. I wouldn't have believed this to be possible a year ago. We all thought women had to have some luteinizing hormone to produce eggs. Now I no longer think that. What does LH do then? I don't know."

In the first six months of 1984, the VIP Program had close to fifty patients being treated with pure FSH alone, about 15 percent of their patients. They were women who had been given Pergonal or a combina-tion of Pergonal with FSH on previous in vitro attempts and did not respond well with these. "Either their estrogen levels did not go up," says Dr. Suheil Muasher, a fellow on the staff, "or we were getting eggs from them that did not fertilize, or we were getting only immature eggs. We stimulated them on a later cycle with only FSH and got much better results. It looks as if we're getting even better quality eggs with pure FSH. Out of these fifty patients, we got eight or nine pregnancies."

The source of the FSH that the Joneses are using is Serono Laborato-ries, which has packaged it under the brand name of Metrodin. However, pure FSH is still in the experimental phase. Until it is approved by the Food and Drug Administration, it is not generally available to other in vitro programs.

When even pure FSH failed to produce follicle growth in one patient in a recent session, the VIP in vitro team refused to acknowledge failure. The patient returned for the next session and a new method of medication was devised for her. An electronic pump about the size of a cigarette package and weighing no more than two ounces was attached to her waist on a belt. From the pump, a thin plastic tube runs up the body and down the arm. At ninety-minute intervals, the pump automatically releases into the patient's arm a gonadotropin releasing hormone which stimulates the pituitary gland to release FSH and LH. (This pump is used in diabetics to administer insulin.) For the first time in five in vitro attempts, this patient's estrogen levels started rising after the first few days of treatment, indicating that there was follicle growth. The estrogen continued to rise and the patient reached the egg retrieval phase. When the in vitro team performed the laparoscopy on this patient, they retrieved one preovulatory oocyte. The egg fertilized and the patient became pregnant. This is the kind of success story that seems to occur at Norfolk on a regular basis.

In addition to modifying the hormone stimulation protocol, the VIP Program has opened its doors to new groups of infertility patients: patients with endometriosis. In the first six months of 1984, the clinic treated twenty-six DES patients, women whose mothers were given the drug DES during their pregnancies to prevent miscarriage. This drug has been found to create infertility in female children. "We've done all right with them," says Dr. Howard Jones, Jr., "six pregnancies out of twenty-six." Norfolk is also now treating infertility patients with immunological problems—antibodies against the husband's sperm—and normal infertile couples. This wide range of patients is a logical outgrowth of the institute's full-service approach to infertility. Not only does The Howard and Georgeanna Jones Institute provide in vitro services, but it also provides consultation and treatment for the whole spectrum of infertility problems.

It is inevitable that as the VIP Program becomes more successful in achieving pregnancies, the applications to the program will continue to rise. The clinic already has over 10,000 applications on file. In response, the Institute has increased its staff and expanded the number of patients it treats each year. In 1984, the Joneses treated 372 patients in five sessions. Half of the patients in each session are new patients. The other half are patients who have failed to get pregnant in previous attempts and come back to try again. Still, no patients in recent cycles have reported any difficulty in being accepted in the VIP Program.

One reason is that many of the 10,000 applicants are not medically viable candidates for the in vitro method. Another factor that eliminates many applicants is that they fail to provide complete medical records, which the application form specifically states is required. The office staff in Norfolk is too small to be able to notify patients when medical records in their applications are incomplete. One patient from North Carolina mailed her application and when she hadn't heard anything after six months, she and her husband made a visit to the Medical Tower office on their next vacation. It turned out that her hysterosalpingogram had never arrived. That was the only thing holding up her application. When she got home, she sent the X-ray to Norfolk by express mail and she was accepted for the next in vitro session.

But it is also because the office staff is small that a telephone call to Linda Lynch is often the most valuable thing an applicant can do on her own behalf. "It's true," says Dr. Howard Jones, Jr. "Whoever screams the loudest to Linda Lynch gets accepted." "They have to be nice about it, though," says Linda Lynch. "I can usually tell by talking to people if they have what it takes to go through the in vitro process."

The cost of the in vitro attempt is another factor that eliminates many applicants. As of January 1985, the cost of one in vitro trial was $4,833, not including transportation, room, and board. Many couples have applied with the expectation that by the time they are accepted, the insurance companies will have decided to cover in vitro fertilization. A few Blue Cross and Blue Shield policies do cover it now. Other insurance companies which do are Banker's Life, Prudential, John Hancock, and Traveler's. Some insurance companies cover in vitro only with expensive special plans.

The Institute cannot subsidize any patients. It is completely fee supported. It receives no funding or grants from any institution or governmental agency. A 1974 federal regulation prohibits the use of federal funds for research in in vitro fertilization in human beings because it is considered an experimental procedure, despite the fact that the Health and Human Services Department affirmed the ethics of in vitro in 1979.

One way the VIP Program is trying to help defray the patients' costs is by planning to convert a nurses' residence on the grounds of the Eastern Virginia Medical School into suites with kitchens for in vitro patients. The funding for this project is being raised privately.

It is clear that as the numbers of patients increase, the individualized approach, which the Joneses feel is the crucial factor in the success of in vitro, becomes much more difficult to maintain. "There is no conceivable way," says Dr. Howard Jones, Jr., "that our program can expand to take care of the demand. It's impossible. We therefore would like to accept the responsibility of improving the success of the in vitro technique in an academic capacity, rather than in a completely clinical capacity. We want to be able to develop to the fullest extent the research potential which lies in our program."

One of the areas in which the Jones Institute is focusing its research efforts is on the aspects of human reproduction about which little is known. No one knows why or how an embryo implants in the uterus. "If we could discover what it is that makes the uterine wall susceptible to implantation," says Dr. Howard Jones, Jr., "we could eliminate the greatest obstacle to the success of in vitro fertilization. We might be able to boost our pregnancy rate to as high as 60 percent."

Another area in which Norfolk is engaged in extensive research is the male factor—the failure of sperm to fertilize an egg. In the institute's Andrology Laboratory, Dr. Stephen Ackerman and his researchers are analyzing sperm to determine the qualities of viable sperm and looking for ways to beef up poor-quality sperm for in vitro fertilization. They have discovered that hyperactivated motility is correlated with the sperm's ability to penetrate an egg. In normal sperm, 2 percent is hyperactivated. In subfertile sperm, hyperactivity is nonexistent.

The researchers found that when they incubated the sperm with poor motility for several hours, they saw an increase in hyperactivated motility. In one sample, 10 percent of the sperm showed hyperactivity as the incubation increased. After four hours' incubation, 40 to 50 percent of the sperm showed hyperactivity. "The longer we incubated the sperm," says Dr. Ackerman, "the more sperm became hyperactive. We've seen samples incubated three to four hours that showed 100 percent hyperactivated motility, but the average is 35 to 50 percent."

"This is a very exciting discovery," says Dr. Howard Jones, Jr. "If we can enhance this quality in our low sperm count group, we can get their eggs fertilized. Once we get fertilization and we go to transfer, then the pregnancy rate for these couples is as good as it is for others."

The result of the Joneses' clinical experience with in vitro fertilization and the research they have conducted toward improving the pregnancy rate has created what Dr. Jones considers to be a unique opportunity for the scientist to examine the process of human reproduction. "What we have learned is that not all of the eggs we retrieve, nor the embryos that we transfer, are of equal potential, and there is no way of determining their potential by looking at them under the microscope. Our efforts so far at the Institute have been dedicated to equalizing the potential of the eggs and the conceptus. Whether this will be successful is very much in doubt because we may be dealing with an inherent problem in human reproduction.

"When you consider the fact," continues Dr. Jones, "that among couples who eventually have a child, the possibility of becoming pregnant in any one month's exposure is less than 25 percent, the question is: What happens to the other 75 percent? In the process of in vitro fertilization, for the first time in history we are able to look at this phenomenon under high power, and what we see are the embryos that in fact are not going to survive. And that's why our results, our pregnancy rates, are as they are. We, like any normal fertile couple, are dealing with this inherent inefficiency of human reproduction.

"This has great significance biologically as well as socially. An understanding of this inefficiency would enable us to improve our efficiency in achieving pregnancy, but it might also make it possible to increase the *in*efficiency of human reproduction. If we could increase the inefficiency of reproduction, we could create a method of birth control that would focus on this factor alone. It would be the equivalent of suppressing fertility with a rifle, a single shot, instead of a shotgun as it is now being done. That's one of the Institute's future objectives."

To explore this objective and other scientific questions about human reproduction, the Joneses have this year added a Basic Science Laboratory to the Institute's other facilities, under the direction of Gary D. Hodgen, Ph.D., the former director of pregnancy research at the National Institutes of Health. Using 250 monkeys, Hodgen will study the underlying causes of infertility and develop new ways to treat them. "We will look at these things in primates first," says Dr. Jones. "Then if they work, use them in our therapeutic work." Hodgen's first priority is to study the "viable embryo factor." "We've got to find a way to identify the embryos that have the highest chance of implantation so that we can maximize our efforts," says Dr. Jones.

Other objectives for the Institute in the future involve the freezing of embryos. Eggs retrieved from a patient during her laparoscopy can be fertilized and then frozen, and saved for transfer to the patient's uterus on a later menstrual cycle when the woman's body has rid itself of the effects of the hormone stimulation and the surgery and anesthesia which might hamper implantation. The advantage of this idea is that a few of these embryos could be used at a time. When one attempt to achieve pregnancy fails in these patients, embryos frozen at the time of the egg retrieval could be used on successive in vitro attempts, without the need for the costly and physically debilitating laparoscopic surgery each time.

Another area that the Jones Institute is developing is a program for donor eggs. "Since we're getting so many eggs now with our FSH protocol, it is not uncommon to get ten," says Dr. Howard Jones, Jr., "we no longer transfer all the eggs. Six is the maximum we will transfer. We have to consider our patients. While multiple births are still rare, we would not want a patient to give birth to more than six babies. Therefore, what becomes of these other eggs?" With a patient's permission, some of her eggs could become donor eggs. A woman who has an infertility problem that prevents her from producing her own eggs could avail herself of these eggs. They would be fertilized by her husband's sperm in a petri dish, implanted in her own uterus, and she would carry the baby to term.

The Joneses, however, have no intention of getting into the business of surrogate mothering. Nor are they interested in pursuing the method developed at UCLA in Torrance, California, in which a fertile woman, capable of producing eggs, is artificially inseminated with sperm from the husband of an infertile woman. When the egg fertilizes, the resulting embryo is then flushed from the body of the fertile woman and implanted in the uterus of the infertile woman. "Asking a woman to have a pregnancy for someone else, even though it is of short duration, is not the same thing as asking a woman to donate an egg retrieved by laparoscopy during an in vitro attempt," says Dr. Georgeanna Jones. "What happens if the embryo fails to be flushed out of the donor's body? That woman is pregnant."

As the new in vitro technology develops, more and more questions like these arise, challenging moral and ethical standards and posing legal dilemmas, none of which are easily resolved. But for Nan and Todd Tilton, there was no moral or legal dilemma. For them in vitro fertilization was, quite simply, a miracle.

The reality now of this miracle is a bit overwhelming sometimes. When Nan looks into the dining room where she used to spread out her wall calendars and plan her life, there are children's toys. She laughs to think how long it's been since she laid out her life so far in advance. Heather and Todd are building a block tower together in an unusual moment of cooperation. Nan holds her breath—at the tenuousness of the tower and the existence of her children. "They're so beautiful, so perfect," says Nan. "It's almost too much. It makes me feel guilty. So many of the in vitro women didn't get pregnant, and I got two, *two babies.*"

The Norfolk in vitro team wants to know when the Tiltons are coming back for a little brother or sister for the twins. "We've got the pattern of response now that works with the Tiltons," says Dr. Howard Jones, Jr.

"We should be able to repeat our success." But Nan and Todd feel that it would be tempting fate. "That's asking too much," says Nan.

Nan has not forgotten the promise she made to God the night before her pregnancy test in the solitude of her hotel room in Norfolk: to be charitable to other people. "My job now," says Nan, "is to help other women get the information they need to find out if in vitro fertilization can work for them."

Down in Norfolk in vitro patients wait in Room 304 at Medical Tower for their daily injections and exams. On the coffee table along with the dog-eared magazines, there is a photograph album, bound in red print gingham and white lace rickrack. On the first page is a photograph of Elizabeth Carr, the first baby conceived by in vitro fertilization to be born in the United States. Below it is a photograph of Heather and Todd Tilton, the country's first in vitro twins. On the following pages are photographs of all the babies that have been born through the Institute's VIP Program.

The photograph album is still far from filled. In the back, in the empty pages where photographs will go, there are scraps of paper, different sizes and shapes and colors, some boldly inscribed, others tentatively. They say, "This space reserved for Baby Houghton"; "This space reserved for Baby Weinstein"; "This space reserved for Baby Collins . . ."

"Our book," says Nan Tilton, "is for these women, women like me who need a miracle."

Appendix A

In Vitro Fertilization Programs in the United States and the World

The following list of facilities is reported to be accepting referrals and/or actively engaged in in vitro fertilization.

This list is for information *only* and does not imply endorsement by The American Fertility Society.

The American Fertility Society cannot attest to the effectiveness of any listed program nor to the completeness of this list.

Also please see Appendix B, "Minimal Standards for Programs of In Vitro Fertilization," established by The American Fertility Society. You may wish to inquire whether the program you are considering meets these standards.

For further information, please contact The American Fertility Society, 2131 Magnolia Avenue, Suite 201, Birmingham, Alabama 35256; (205) 251-9764

Rev: 1/11/85

IN VITRO FERTILIZATION PROGRAMS

ALABAMA

University of Alabama-Birmingham Medical Center
Laboratory for IVF-ET
547 Old Hillman Building, University Station
Birmingham, AL 35294
(205) 934-5631
Director: Kathryn L. Honea, M.D.

ARIZONA

Phoenix Fertility Institute P.C.
(Good Samaritan Hospital)
1300 North 12th Street, Suite 522
Phoenix, AZ 85006
Director: Tawfik H. Rizkallah, M.D.

CALIFORNIA

Alta Bates Hospital
In Vitro Fertilization Program
3001 Colby Street
Berkeley, CA 94705
(415) 540-1416
Director: Ryszard J. Chetkowski, M.D.

Fertility Institute of San Diego
(Sharp/Children's Medical Center)
9834 Genessee Avenue, Suite 300
La Jolla, CA 92037
(619) 455-7520
Director: Joseph F. Kennedy, M.D.
Contact: Susan Abbott

Scripps Clinic and Research Foundation (PRIVATE)
10666 North Torrey Pines Road
La Jolla, CA 92037
(619) 457-8680

Beverly Hills Medical Center
Department of Ob/Gyn
1177 South Beverly Drive
Los Angeles, CA 90024

University of Southern California School of Medicine
IVF-Embryo Replacement Program
Hospital of the Good Samaritan
637 South Lucas Avenue
Los Angeles, CA 90017
(213) 226-3421
Director: Richard Marrs, M.D., Joyce Vargyas, M.D.

Southern California Fertility Institute (PRIVATE)
12301 Wilshire Boulevard, Suite 415
Los Angeles, CA 90025
Director: William Karow, M.D.

Century City Hospital
2070 Century Park East
Los Angeles, CA 90067
(213) 201-6619
Director: Dianne Moore Smith, Ph.D.

Northridge Hospital Medical Center
IVF Program
18300 Roscoe Boulevard
Northridge, CA 91328
(818) 996-2289
Director: Sheldon L. Schein, M.D., and Paul M. Greenberg, M.D.

University of California, San Francisco
IVF Program
Department of Ob/Gyn & Reproductive Sciences
Room M 1480
San Francisco, CA 94143
(415) 666-1824
Director: Robert H. Glass, M.D., and Mary C. Martin, M.D.
Contact: Marion Wiener

UCLA-Harbor
Department of Ob/Gyn
1000 West Carson D-3
Torrance, CA 90509

John Muir Memorial Hospital
Department of Ob/Gyn: IVF Program
Walnut Creek, CA 94598
(415) 937-6166
Director: Donald Galen, M.D., Arnold Jacobson, M.D., and Elwood Kronick,
    M.D.

CANADA

University of Calgary
In Vitro Fertilization Program
3330 Hospital Drive N.W.
Calgary, *Alberta*
Canada T2N 4N1
(403) 283-7531
Director: P. J. Taylor, M.D.
NOTE: Alberta residents only

University of British Columbia
Grace Hospital
Department of Ob/Gyn
4490 Oak Street
Vancouver, *British Columbia*
Canada V6H 3V5

Dalhousie University
IVF Programme
c/o Endocrine and Infertility Centre
5821 University Avenue
Halifax, *Nova Scotia*
Canada B3H 1W3
Director: William Wrixon, M.D.

University Hospital
University of Western Ontario
In Vitro Fertilization Program
339 Windermere Road
London, *Ontario*
Canada N6A 5A5
(519) 663-2966
Director: A. A. Yuzpe, M.D.
Contact: Mrs. Heather Erskine

Toronto East General Hospital
LIFE Program
825 Coxwell Avenue
Toronto, *Ontario*
Canada M4C 3G2

Le Centre Hospitalier de l'Université Laval
La consultation de Fertilité, F.E.C.
2705 Boulevard Laurier
Ste. Foy, *Quebec*
Canada G1V 4G2
(418) 656-8197
Director: Jacques E. Rioux, M.D.
Contact: Rita Richard, R.N.

COLORADO

University of Colorado Health Sciences Center
IVF Program
4200 East 9th Avenue, Box B198
Denver, CO 80262
(303) 394-8365
Director: Bruce H. Albrecht, M.D.
Contact: Rhonda Holloway, R.N., Clinical Coordinator

Reproductive Genetics In Vitro PC (PRIVATE)
6445 East Ohio Avenue, Suite 500
Denver, CO 80224
(303) 399-1464
Director: George Henry, M.D.

CONNECTICUT

University of Connecticut Health Center
Division of Reproductive Endocrinology & Infertility
Farmington, CT 06790
(203) 674-2110
Director: Daniel H. Riddick, M.D., Ph.D.
Contact: Helene Clyburn

Mount Sinai Hospital
Department of Ob/Gyn: Division of Reproductive Endocrinology and
    Infertility
675 Hartford Avenue
Hartford, CT 06112
(203) 242-6201
Director: Augusto P. Chong, M.D.

Yale University Medical School
Department of Ob/Gyn: IVF Program
333 Cedar Street
New Haven, CT 06510
(203) 785-4019, 785-4792
Director: Alan DeCherney, M.D.

DISTRICT OF COLUMBIA

Columbia Hospital for Women Medical Center
IVF Program
2425 L. Street NW
Washington, D.C. 20037
(202) 293-6500
Director: Richard Falk, M.D.
Contact: Sheri Schlafstein, R.N.

George Washington University Medical Center
Department of Ob/Gyn: IVF Program
901 23rd Street N.W.
Washington, D.C. 20037
(202) 676-4614
Director: Robert J. Stillman, M.D.

FLORIDA

University of Miami
Department of Ob/Gyn: D-5
P. O. Box 016960
Miami, FL 33101
(305) 547-5818
Director: T. T. Hung, M.D., Ph.D

GEORGIA

Atlanta Center for Fertility and Endocrinology
(Northside Hospital)
5675 Peachtree-Dunwoody Road N.E.
Atlanta, GA 30342
(404) 256-8000
Director: Camran Nezhat, M.D.

Atlanta Fertility Institute
(Georgia Baptist Medical Center)
300 Boulevard N.E.
Atlanta, GA 30312
(404) 659-5211
Director: Amir H. Ansari, M.D.

Reproductive Biology Associates (PRIVATE)
993F Johnson Ferry Road, Suite 240
Atlanta, GA 30342
(404) 252-1137
Director: Hilton Kort, M.D., Joe Massey, M.D.

Augusta Reproductive Biology Associates (PRIVATE)
810-812 Chafee
Augusta, GA 30904

Medical College of Georgia
Humana Hospital-IVF Section
Augusta, GA 30912
Director: Paul McDonough, M.D.

HAWAII

Kapiolani Children's Hospital
Department of Ob/Gyn
1319 Punahou Street
Honolulu, HI 96826
Director: Thomas T. F. Huang, M.D.

ILLINOIS

University of Illinois College of Medicine
Department of Ob/Gyn
840 South Wood Street
Chicago, IL 60612

Michael Reese-University of Chicago
IVF-ET Program
31st Street at Lake Shore Drive
Chicago, IL 60616
(312) 791-4000
Director: Edward L. Marut, M.D.
Contact: Mary Coppolillo, Coordinator

Mount Sinai Hospital Medical Center
Department of Ob/Gyn: IVF Program
California Avenue at 15th Street
Chicago, IL 60608
(312) 650-6727
Director: Norbert Gleicher, M.D., Jan Friberg, M.D.

Rush Medical College
IVF Program: Department of Ob/Gyn
600 South Paulina Street
Chicago, IL 60616
(312) 942-6609
Director: W. Paul Dmowski, M.D., Ph.D.

INDIANA

Indiana University Medical Center
Department of Ob/Gyn: Section of Reproductive Endocrinology
926 West Michigan Street, N. 262
Indianapolis, IN 46223
(317) 264-4057
Director: Marguerite K. Shepard, M.D.

KANSAS

Kansas University Gynecological & Obstetrical Foundation
University of Kansas College of Health Sciences
39th Street and Rainbow Boulevard
Kansas City, KS 66103
(913) 588-6246
Director: William J. Cameron, M.D.
Contact: Peggy Everly

KENTUCKY

University of Kentucky Medical College
Department of Ob/Gyn
Lexington, KY 40536

Norton Hospital
IVF Program
610 South Floyd Street
Louisville, KY 40202
(502) 583-3845
Director: Marvin A. Yussman, M.D.
Contact: Susan Beatty, R.N., Coordinator

LOUISIANA

The Fertility Institute of New Orleans
(Pendleton Memorial Methodist Hospital)
9830 Lake Forest Boulevard, Suite 118
New Orleans, LA 70127
Director: Richard Dickey, M.D.
Contact: Susie White, Coordinator

Tulane University
IVF Program
Department of Ob/Gyn
1430 Tulane Avenue
New Orleans, LA 70112
Director: Ian H. Thorneycroft, M.D.

MARYLAND

Baltimore IVF Clinic (PRIVATE)
2435 West Belvedere Avenue #41
Baltimore, MD 21215

Greater Baltimore Medical Center (PRIVATE)
IVF Program of the Women's Fertility Center
6701 North Charles Street
Baltimore, MD 21204
(301) 828-2484
Director: Frederick Weinstein, M.D.
Contact: Sue Meeks, Coordinator

The Johns Hopkins Hospital
Division of Reproductive Endocrinology: IVF Program
600 North Wolfe Street
Baltimore, MD 21205
Director: John A. Rock, M.D.
Contact: Marion Damewood, M.D.

Union Memorial Hospital
IVF Program: Department of Ob/Gyn
201 East University Parkway
Baltimore, MD 21218
(301) 235-5255
Director: Rafael Haciski, M.D.

Genetic Consultants
(Washington Adventist Hospital)
5616 Shields Drive
Bethesda, MD 20817
(301) 530-6900
Director: Mark Geier, M.D., John Young, M.D.
Contact: Janet Rodenhiser, R.N.

MASSACHUSETTS

Beth Israel Hospital
Department of Ob/Gyn: IVF Program
330 Brookline Avenue
Boston, MA 02215
Director: Melvin Taymor, M.D., Machelle Seibel, M.D.

Brigham and Womens Hospital
IVF Program
75 Francis Street
Boston, MA 02115
Director: Daniel Tulchinsky, M.D.
Contact: Debby Carnes, Administrative Secretary

Tufts-New England Medical Center
Department of Ob/Gyn: Division of Reproductive Endocrinology
171 Harrison Avenue
Boston, MA 02111

Greater Boston In Vitro Associates (PRIVATE)
(Newton-Wellesley Hospital)
2000 Washington Street, Suite 342
Newton, Ma 02162
(617) 965-7270
Director: John H. Derry, M.D., Peter M. Martin, M.D., Robert A. Newton,
    M.D., Director of Andrology
Contact: Roberta Hayes, R.N., Coordinator

MICHIGAN

University of Michigan Medical Center
L-2120 Women's Hospital
Department of Ob/Gyn
Ann Arbor, MI 48109
(313) 763-4323
Director: Jonathan Ayers, M.D.
Contact: Ann N. Brown, R.N., Coordinator

Blodgett Memorial Medical Center
IVF Program
1900 Wealthy Street S.E., Suite 330
Grand Rapids, MI 49506
(616) 774-0700
Director: Robert D. Visscher, M.D.
Contact: Mary Hager

Hutzel Hospital/Wayne State University
IVF Program
4707 St. Antoine Street
Detroit, MI 48201
(313) 494-7547
Director: David M. Magyar, D.O.
Contact: Patricia Rogers, R.N., Clinical Coordinator

William Beaumont Hospital
In Vitro Fertilization Program
3601 West 13 Mile Road
Royal Oak, MI 48072
(313) 288-2380
Director: S. Jan Behrman, M.D.
Contact: Deborah Venettis, R.N., CNC

MINNESOTA

University of Minnesota VIP Program
Department of Ob/Gyn
Box 395, Mayo Memorial Building
420 Delaware Street S.E.
Minneapolis, MN 55455
(612) 373-8852
Director: George Tagatz, M.D.
Contact: Kay F. Riviello

Mayo Clinic
Department of Reproductive Endocrinology & Infertility
200 First Street S.W.
Rochester, MN 55905
(507) 284-3188
Director: Carolyn B. Coulam, M.D.
Contact: Cammy Kelley, Fertility Clinic Coordinator

MISSISSIPPI

University of Mississippi Medical Center
IVF Program
Department of Ob/Gyn
Jackson, MS 39216
(601) 987-4662
Director: Bryan D. Cowan, M.D.
Contact: Susan Jarvis

MISSOURI

Jewish Hospital
Department of Ob/Gyn: IVF Program
216 South Kings Highway
St. Louis, MO 63110
Director: Ronald Strickler, M.D.
Contact: Cat Christianson, R.N.

Missouri Baptist Hospital
In Vitro Fertilization Program, Room 301
3015 North Ballas Road
St. Louis, MO 63131
(314) 432-1212, Ext. 5295
Director: Romeo Perez, M.D.
Contact: Patricia Bircher, R.N., Coordinator

NEBRASKA

University of Nebraska Medical Center
Department of Ob/Gyn
42nd Street and Dewey Avenue
Omaha, NE 68105
(402) 559-4212
Director: Raymond Schulte, M.D.
Contact: Margaret Christiansen, R.N.

NEVADA

Northern Nevada Fertility Clinic (PRIVATE)
350 West 6th Street
Reno, NV 89503
(702) 322-4521
Director: Geoffrey Sher, M.D.

NEW JERSEY

New Jersey School of Osteopathic Medicine
JFK-Cherry Hill Division
Department of Ob/Gyn
Cherry Hill, NJ 08034

University Hospital
Department of Ob/Gyn
100 Bergen Street
Newark, NJ 07103

UMD: Rutgers Medical School
Department of Ob/Gyn: IVF Program
Academic Health Science Center, CN19
New Brunswick, NJ 08903
(201) 937-7635
Director: Ekkehard Kemmann, M.D.

NEW YORK

Childrens Hospital
Reproduction and Infertility Unit
IVF-ET Program
140 Hodge Avenue
Buffalo, NY 14222

Mount Sinai Medical Center
In Vitro Fertilization Program
One Gustave Levy Place
Annenberg 20-60
New York, NY 10029
Director: Jon W. Gordon, M.D., Ph.D.
Contact: Debra Sperling, R.N., Coordinator

North Shore University Hospital
Division of Human Reproduction: IVF
300 Community Drive
Manhasset, NY 11030
(516) 562-4470
Director: Richard Bronson, M.D.
Contact: Rise Weinberg, R.N.

Columbia-Presbyterian Medical Center
Presbyterian Hospital IVF-ET Program
622 West 168th Street
New York, NY 10032
(212) 694-8013
Director: Georgianna Jagiello, M.D.
Contact: Elynne B. Margulis, M.D., Medical Coordinator

University of Rochester CARE Program
University of Rochester Medical Center
Rochester, NY 14642
(716) 275-4422
Director: Eberhard Muechler, M.D.

NORTH CAROLINA

North Carolina Memorial Hospital
Fertility Center: IVF Program
Chapel Hill, NC 27514
(919) 966-5438
Director: Luther M. Talbert, M.D.
Contact: Linda Bailey, R.N., Nurse Coordinator

Chapel Hill Fertility Services (PRIVATE)
109 Conner Drive, Suite 2104
Chapel Hill, NC 27514
Director: James Dingfeld, M.D.

Duke University Medical Center
Department of Ob/Gyn: IVF Program
P. O. Box 3143, DUMC
Durham, NC 27710
(919) 684-5327
Director: James F. Holman, M.D.

OHIO

Jewish Hospital
Department of Ob/Gyn: IVF Program
3120 Burnet Avenue
Cincinnati, OH 45229

University of Cincinnati Medical Center
IVF Program
Division of Reproductive Endocrinology & Infertility
Department of Ob/Gyn
231 Bethesda Avenue
Cincinnati, OH 45267
(513) 872-6368
Director: O'dell M. Owens, M.D.
Contact: Jan Hill, R.N.

Cleveland Clinic Foundation
In Vitro Fertilization Program
9500 Euclid Avenue
Cleveland, OH 44106
(216) 444-2240
Director: Martin M. Quigley, M.D.

MacDonald Hospital for Women
IVF Program
2105 Adelbert Road
Cleveland, OH 44106
Director: J. DeFazio, M.D.

Mount Sinai Medical Center of Cleveland
LIFE Program
University Circle
Cleveland, OH 44106
(216) 421-5884
Director: Wulf H. Utian, M.D.

University Reproductive Center
Ohio State University Hospitals
410 West 10th Avenue
Columbus, OH 43210
(614) 421-8937, 421-8511
Director: Moon H. Kim, M.D.
Contact: Mrs. Virginia Christman

Infertility and Gynecology, Inc.
(Grant Hospital)
1450 Hawthorne Avenue
Columbus, OH 43203
(614) 253-8383
Director: Nichols Vorys, M.D.
Contact: Barbara Foor, R.N.

Miami Valley Hospital
In Vitro Fertilization Program
1 Wyoming Street
Dayton, OH 45409
(513) 223-6192, Ext. 4066
Director: Robert C. Winslow, M.D.
Contact: Valerie Upshaw, R.N.

OKLAHOMA

Hillcrest Infertility Center
1145 South Utica, #1209
Tulsa, OK 74104
(918) 584-2870
Director: J. Clark Bundron, M.D., J. W. Edward Wortham, Ph.D.
Contact: Kay Smittle

OREGON

Oregon Reproductive Research & Fertility Program
Oregon Health Science University School of Medicine
3181 S.W. Sam Jackson Park Road
Portland, OR 97201
(503) 225-8449
Director: Kenneth A. Burry, M.D.

PENNSYLVANIA

Hospital of the University of Pennsylvania
Department of Ob/Gyn: IVF Program
3400 Spruce Street, Suite 106
Philadelphia, PA 19104
(215) 662-2981
Director: Luigi Mastroianni, Jr., M.D., Celso-Ramon Garcia, M.D.
Program Coordinator: Richard Tureck, M.D.

The Pennsylvania Hospital
In Vitro Fertilization-Embryo Transfer Program
Eighth & Spruce Streets
Philadelphia, PA 19107
Director: Esther Eisenberg, M.D.
Contact: Mary English, R.N., Coordinator

Magee-Women's Hospital
IVF Program
Forbes Avenue and Halket Street
Pittsburgh, PA 15213
(412) 647-4000
Director: Paul Zarutski, M.D.

SOUTH CAROLINA

Medical University of South Carolina
Department of Ob/Gyn: IVF Program
171 Ashley Avenue
Charleston, SC 29425
Director: Charles Tsai, M.D.

The Southeastern Fertility Center
(Roper Hospital)
315 Calhoun Street
Charleston, SC 29401
(803) 722-3294
Director: Grant Patton, M.D., John Black, Ph.D.
Contact: Margaret Moxley, Program Coordinator

TENNESSEE

East Tennessee Baptist Hospital
Family Life Center
7A Office 715
Box 1788, Blount Avenue
Knoxville, TN 37901
Director: I. Ray King, M.D.
Contact: Linda Pendergrass

University of Tennessee Memorial Research Center and Hospital
1924 Alcoa Highway
Knoxville, TN 37920
(615) 971-4958
Director: Robert A. Wild, M.D.
Contact: Michael R. Caudle, M.D., Coordinator, Debra Rose, R.N.

Vanderbilt University
In Vitro Fertilization Program
D3200 Medical Center North
Nashville, TN 37232
(615) 322-6576
Director: Anne Colston Wentz, M.D.
Contact: Catherine H. Garner, R.N.

TEXAS

St. David's Community Hospital
In Vitro Fertilization-ET Program
P. O. Box 4039 (919 East 32nd Street)
Austin, TX 78765
(512) 397-4107, 476-7111
Director: Thomas Vaughn, M.D.
Contact: Ruby Diane Fischer, R.N.C., Coordinator

Lutheran Medical System North/Texas
Carrollton Community Hospital
1711 South Broadway
Carrollton, TX 75006
(214) 245-5983, 245-5984
Director: W. F. "Dub" Howard, M.D.
Contact: Alice Polakoff, R.N.

Presbyterian Hospital of Dallas
P. O. Box 17 (8160 Walnut Hill Lane)
Dallas, TX 75231
(214) 891-2624
Director: James D. Madden, M.D.
Contact: Judy Newby, R.N.

University of Texas HSC-Dallas
Department of Ob/Gyn
5303 Harry Hines Boulevard
Dallas, TX 75235

Fort Worth Reproductive Center (PRIVATE)
1050 Fifth Avenue, Suite A
Fort Worth, TX 76109

University of Texas Medical Branch
Department of Ob/Gyn: IVF Program
Galveston, TX 77550
(409) 761-3985
Director: Manubai Nagamani, M.D.

Baylor College of Medicine
Department of Ob/Gyn: IVF Program
1 Baylor Plaza
Houston, TX 77030

Texas Woman's Hospital
IVF Program
7600 Fannin Street
Houston, TX 77054

Sam Houston IVF Centre (PRIVATE)
1615 Hillendahl Boulevard
Houston, TX 77055

University of Texas Health Science Center
Department of Ob/Gyn & Reproductive Science
6431 Fannin Street, Suite 3270
Houston, TX 77030
(713) 792-5360
Director: Pedro Beauchamp, M.D., Donald P. Wolf, Ph.D.
Contact: Marjorie Stringer

Texas Tech University School of Medicine
Department of Ob/Gyn
P. O. Box 4569
Lubbock, TX 79409

University of Texas Health Science Center
Department of Ob/Gyn: IVF Program
7703 Floyd Curl Drive
San Antonio, TX 78284
Director: Ricardo Asch, M.D.

Texas A&M University
Scott and White Medical Center
Department of Ob/Gyn
Temple, TX 76508

UTAH

University of Utah
Division of Reproductive Endocrinology
50 Medical Drive North
Salt Lake City, UT 84132
(801) 581-4837
Director: William Keye, M.D.

VIRGINIA

Fairfax-Northern Virginia Genetics & IVF Institute
(Fairfax Hospital)
3020 Javier Road
Fairfax, VA 22031
(703) 469-9530
Director: Joseph D. Schulman, M.D.

Eastern Virginia Medical School
Jones Institute for Reproductive Medicine
304 Medical Tower
Norfolk, VA 23507
(804) 628-3370
Director: Howard W. Jones, Jr., M.D., Georgeanna Seegar Jones, M.D.

Medical College of Virginia
IVF Program
Box 34—MCV Station
Richmond, VA 23298
(804) 786-9636
Director: Sanford M. Rosenberg, M.D.
Contact: Robin Doran

WASHINGTON

Swedish Hospital Medical Center
Reproductive Genetics
747 Summit Avenue
Seattle, WA 98104
(206) 292-2483
Director: Laurence E. Karp, M.D.
Contact: Dianne Smith, Associate Director

University of Washington IVF Program
Department of Ob/Gyn: RH-20
Seattle, WA 98195
(206) 543-8483
Director: Michael Soules, M.D.
Contact: Pattei Lazear, C.R.N., Cindy Schuler

WISCONSIN

University of Wisconsin Clinics
IVF Program
600 Highland Avenue
H4/630 CSC
Madison, WI 53792
(608) 263-1217
Director: Sander S. Shapiro, M.D.
Contact: Janet Slowinski, Program Coordinator

University of WI-Milwaukee Clinical Campus
Department of Ob/Gyn
Mount Sinai Medical Center
950 North 12th Street
P. O. Box 342
Milwaukee, WI 53201
(414) 289-8609
Director: Mark R. Neff, M.D.
Contact: Margaret Nicoud, Nurse Coordinator

Milwaukee Regional Fertility Center
IVF Program
426 West Main Street
Waukesha, WI 53186

AUSTRALIA

Monash University Medical School
Queen Victoria Hospital
Department of Ob/Gyn
172 Lonsdale Street
Melbourne, Victoria, Australia 3000
Director: Alan Trounson, M.D.

University of Melbourne
Royal Womens Hospital
Department of Ob/Gyn
Melbourne, Victoria, Australia
Director: Alexander Lopata, M.D.

Lingard Hospital
In Vitro Fertilization Programme
Merewether, Newcastle NSW Australia 2291
049 696799
Director: J. D. Stanger, M.D.
Coordinator: M. Oliver

Royal North Shore Hospital of Sydney
Department of Ob/Gyn
St Leonards NSW Australia
(02) 438 7027
Director: Douglas M. Saunders, M.D.

King Edward Memorial Hospital
University Department of Ob/Gyn
Bagot Road
Subiaco 6008 Western Australia
(09) 382 1677
Director: John L. Yovich, M.D.

Westmead Centre
Parramatta Hospitals
IVF Program
Sydney, Australia 2000

Cambridge Hospital
PIVET Laboratory
178 Cambridge Street
Wembley 6014 Western Australia
Director: John L. Yovich, M.D.

AUSTRIA

Fertility Centre
Formanekgasse 57
1190 *Vienna* Austria
Director: Peter Hernuss, M.D.

Institute of Reproductive Endocrinology and In Vitro Fertilization
Trauttmansdorffgasse 3A
1130 *Vienna* Austria
Director: Peter Kemeter, M.D., Wilfried Feichtinger, M.D.

BELGIUM

University of Leuven
Gasthuisberg University Hospital
Department of Ob/Gyn
Leuven, Belgium
Director: P. R. Koninekx, M.D.

COLOMBIA

Cecolfes
Centro Colombiano de Fertilidad y Esterilidad
Calle 93A #10-55
Bogota, Colombia

ENGLAND

Bourne Hall Clinic
Bourne, Cambridge CB3 7TR England
Medical Director: Patrick Steptoe, M.D.
Scientific Director: Robert G. Edwards, Ph.D.

Rosie Maternity Hospital
Department of Ob/Gyn
Cambridge CB2 2SW England

In Vitro Fertilization Clinic
25 Weymouth Street
London W1 England

John Radcliffe Hospital
Nuffield Department of Ob/Gyn
IVF Programme
Oxford OX3 9AY England

Princess Anne Hospital
University of Southampton
Department of Human Reproduction & Ob
Coxford Road
Southampton S09 4HA England
Director: Gordon Masson, M.D.

FRANCE

The American Hospital of Paris
IVF Program
63 Boulevard Victor Hugo
92202 *Neuilly Sur Seine*
France
747 5300
Director: Jacques Testart, M.D.
Contact: Bruce Redor

Hôpital Tenon
Department of Ob/Gyn
4 Rue de la Grave
Paris
France
Director: Jacques Salat-Baroux, M.D.
Contact: Jacqueline Mandelbaum

HONG KONG

Chinese University of Hong Kong
Department of Ob/Gyn
Shatin, New Territory
Hong Kong

ISRAEL

Hadassah University Hospital
Department of Reproductive Medicine
P. O. Box 12000
91120 *Jerusalem* Israel

Sheba Medical Center
Department of Reproductive Medicine
52621 *Tel Hashomer* Israel

ITALY

FIV/ET Programme
54 Via Villareale
90100 *Palermo,* Italy
Director: Annele Battaglia, M.D.

Gruppo FIV-ET, Torino
Istituto di Ginecologia dell'Universita
  e Ospedale Sant'Anna
Via Ventimiglia 1
10126 *Torino* Italy
011/6563
Director: Professor Carlo Campagnoli, Alessandro DiGregorio, M.D., Riccardo
  Arisio, M.D.

JAPAN

Fukui Red Cross Hospital
IVF Program
Fukui 910-11 Japan

Dokkyu University
Department of Ob/Gyn
Mibu Tochigi 321-02 Japan

NETHERLANDS

Sint Annadel University Hospital
Department of Ob/Gyn
P. O. Box 1918
6201 BX *Maastricht* Netherlands

University Hospital Dykzigt
Dr Molewaterplein 40
3015 GD *Rotterdam* Netherlands
Director: Alberda, M.D., Zeilmaker, M.D.

SINGAPORE

National University of Singapore
Kandang Kerbau Hospital
Department of Ob/Gyn
Hampshire Road
Singapore 0821 Singapore
Director: Professor S. S. Ratnam

SPAIN

CEFER
c/Mare de Deu de la Salut 78 1 c
08024 *Barcelona* Spain
Director: Luis C. Pous-Ivern, M.D.

SWEDEN

Sahlgrenska University Hospital
Department of Ob/Gyn
S-413 45 *Gothenburg* Sweden
(031) 60 33 38
Contact: Lars Nilsson, M.D., Ph.D.

SWITZERLAND

CHUV
Department of Ob/Gyn
CH-1011 *Lausanne* Switzerland
(021) 41 25 30-411 11
Director: P. De Grandi, M.D.

TAIWAN

Chang Gung Memorial Hospital
IVF-ET Program
199 Tung-Hwa North Road
Taipei Taiwan

Veterans General Hospital
Department of Ob/Gyn
Taipei 112 Taiwan

THAILAND

Chulalongkorn Hospital University
Department of Ob/Gyn
Bangkok Thailand

WEST GERMANY

Auguste-Viktoria Krankenhaus
IVF-Labor Haus 35
Rubensstrasse 125
1000 *Berlin* 45 West Germany

University of Dusseldorf
Department of Ob/Gyn
Moorenstrasse 5
4000 *Dusseldorf* West Germany
Director: Hugo C. Verhoeven, M.D.

Universitats-Frauenklinik Erlangen
Program for Extracorporeal In Vitro Fertilization
Universitatsstrasse 21-23
8520 *Erlangen* West Germany
(9131) 85-4822
Director: Siegfried Trotnow, M.D.
Contact: Tobias L. A. Hunlich, M.D., Peter Habermann, M.D.

Fertility Institute
Kettwiger Strasse 2-10
4300 *Essen* West Germany
Director: Katzorke, M.D., Propping, M.D.

University Hospitals
Department of Ob/Gyn
Hufland Strasse 55
4300 *Essen* 1 West Germany

Appendix B

"Minimal Standards for Programs of
In Vitro Fertilization"

I. General Conclusions

Every group initiating a program of in vitro fertilization should have all aspects of the program approved by a properly constituted Institutional Review Committee. The Institutional Review Committee or its equivalent should ensure that a record is kept of all attempts made at securing pregnancies by these techniques. The records should include all medical aspects of the treatment cycles and a record of success or failure with respect to oocyte recovery, fertilization, cleavage, conceptus transfer, biophysical monitoring of fetal growth, pregnancy outcome, and complications. These institutional records, which should be separate from the regular records of the medical institution, should be confidential. Summaries for statistical purposes, including details of any congenital abnormalities among offspring, should be available for correlation.

It is recommended that special attention be given to the emotional needs and the emotional support of these patients.

It is recommended that the director of the program have clinical experience and competence.

In view of the many research opportunities offered by programs of in vitro fertilization, it is urged that all programs be designed to take advantage of these opportunities.

II. Personnel

Personnel with the following four types of skills are required as a minimum. A single individual may possess one or more of the required skills.

(1) An individual with the experience and training required for board certification in reproductive endocrinology. While individuals with equivalent training and experience are certainly acceptable, board certification

clearly indicates that the required skills in reproductive endocrinology have been obtained.

(2) A pelvic reparative surgeon with laparoscopic experience with evidence of specialized training in follicular aspiration.

(3) An individual experienced in male reproduction (andrology) with special competence in semenology.

(4) An individual with knowledge of and practical experience in tissue culture, gamete maturation, fertilization, and early zygote cleavage in human and animal systems.

III. Special Services and Facilities

These services and facilities must be on call on a daily basis with twenty-four-hour availability.

(1) Ultrasonography.

(2) Hormonal assays.

(3) Facilities for follicular aspiration and conceptus transfer.

(4) Anesthesia.

(5) A laboratory for gamete fertilization and conceptus development near the operating room with two-way communication between the laboratory and operating room.

—Report of an ad hoc committee of The American Fertility Society: Howard W. Jones, Jr., M.D., Chairman, Anne Colston Wentz, M.D., Martin M. Quigley, M.D., Richard P. Marrs, M.D., and C. Alvin Paulsen, M.D. Approved by the Board of Directors of The American Fertility Society.

Index

A

Ackerman, Stephen, 157
Acosta, Anibel, 81, 87, 111–12
"Adopting a sperm," 27
    See also Artificial
        insemination
Adoption, 4, 46, 70
Alcohol use, effect on
        embryonic development,
        83, 118, 129
All in the Family, 121
Amelar, Richard, 19, 23–28, 69
Amelar-Dubin procedure for
        variocele surgery, 24
American Fertility Society,
        The, 2, 152
Amniocentesis, 129
Andrews, Mason, 58, 59, 79–80
Andrology survey, 68
    See also Sperm analysis
Anesthesia, effect on eggs, 77,
        107, 129
Antibiotics, 109
A Pattern of response to
        hormone stimulation, 89
Artificial insemination, 4, 27–
        29, 31–32, 38, 44
    confidentiality concerns, 30,
        37
    cost of, 30
    insurance coverage for, 150
    pregnancy, chance of, 30

sperm donors for, 29–30, 33–
        34
Azospermia, 64

B

Babies
    birth weight of, 138
    buying babies, 4, 46
Basal temperature, 32, 103
Basal temperature chart, 1, 13,
        31, 34
Birth control, research on, 158
Birth control pills, 11
B Pattern of response to
        hormone stimulation, 89
Brown, Lesley, 56, 71, 80, 96
Brown, Louise, 51, 55, 58, 61,
        69, 71, 80, 96
Business Week, 49
Buying babies, 4, 46

C

Caesarian section surgery, 139,
        140, 142–44
    husband's presence during,
        141, 142, 143

Cambridge University
  Bourne Hall, 58, 150
  Physiological Laboratory, 52
Carr, Elizabeth Jordan, 79, 80
Carr, Judy, 65–66, 69–71, 79–80
Carr, Roger, 66, 69–71, 80
Catholic Charities, 38
Cervix, 11–12
  mucus of, 2, 12, 13, 32, 34, 87, 97, 104, 154
Childbearing, postponement of, 3
Child Is Born, A (Nilsson), 123
Children's Hospital of The King's Daughters (Norfolk, Va.), 147
Cilia of fallopian tubes, 12, 42
Clomiphene, 62
Coffee, effect on embryonic development, 83
Coleridge, Jan, 98, 126
Corpus luteum, 13
Crick, Francis, 55
Cumulus, 110
C. W. Post College, 4, 5, 9, 10, 46
Cystoscope, 53

D

Decker, Albert, 53
Delalutin, 129, 133
DES (diethyl stilbestrol) patients, 155
Diaphragms, 11

Doppler (ultrasonic instrument), 135
Doris (nurse in VIP program), 98, 100, 148
Dubin, Lawrence, 19, 24

E

Eastern Virginia Medical School (Norfolk, Va.), 48, 59–60, 69, 145
  See also VIP Program
Eastern Virginia Medical School Foundation, 59
Ectopic pregnancy, 61, 69–70
Edwards, Robert, 45, 51–52, 58, 60, 61, 63, 69, 80, 150, 152
Eggs, 11, 90
  donor eggs, 158–59
  incubation of, 63, 70, 108, 110
  maturity, classification of, 108
  number retrieved, 108, 112, 115, 152
  retrieval process, 56–57, 70, 75–76, 85–86, 90
Ejaculation, 12–13
Ellis, Linda, 98
Embryologist, role in in vitro fertilization, 107–8, 110
Embryos
  development of, factors influencing, 83
  freezing of, 158

implantation in uterus, 157
incubation of, 110
number transferred, 116–17,
    120, 127, 152
transferral process, 57–58,
    70, 117–18, 119–20
"viable embryo factor," 158
Endometriosis, 2, 16–17, 38,
    40, 41, 151, 155
Estrogen, 11, 56, 85, 87
    patterns of response to
        hormone stimulation,
        89, 96
Exercise, effect on embryonic
    development, 83

Fimbria, 12, 42
Follicles, 13
    hormones of, 11, 13
    monitoring of, 84
    ultrasound imaging, 88–89,
        97
Follicle stimulating hormone
    (FSH), 11, 12, 25, 62,
    85–86, 87, 108, 154
Ford Foundation, 52
Frangenheim, Hans, 54
Frank, L. Matthew, 149
Friends Academy, 4, 9, 81, 135
FSH. *See* Follicle stimulating
    hormone

F

G

Fallopian tubes, 12
    blockage of, 37–38, 40, 41–
        44
    cilia of, 12, 42
    removal of, 61
    role of, 42
    scar tissue on, 2, 3, 75–76
    tubal insufflation test, 35
Fenton, Arnold, 131
Fertility drugs, 62
Fertilization, 11, 13
Fetus
    development of, 135–36, 137
    sensitivity of, 138
Fiber optics, 54, 55

Garcia, Jairo, 70, 71, 74–78,
    81, 87, 89–90, 93, 97,
    100–4, 106, 109–14,
    116–17, 119–20, 122,
    124–25, 127–30, 136–
    37, 145, 147–49, 150,
    152, 153
Gilbert, Michael, 142, 145
Gloves, sterile, effect on
        embryos, 117–18
Goldman, Mitchell, 136
Goldstein, Deborah, 22, 40
G Pattern of response to
        hormone stimulation, 89

H

Hams F-10 culture medium, 55
Hanna, Betsy, 106, 112, 119,
    120–21
Having Twins (Noble), 137
HCG. *See* Human chorionic
    gonadotropin
Health Services Administration
    (HSA), 60
Hickock, Doug and Sandra, 22
HMG. *See* Human menopausal
    gonadotropin
Hodgen, Gary D., 158
Hofheimer, Henry Clay, II, 59
Hormone injection, side effects
    of, 92, 96, 100
Hormones
    female, 11–12, 56
    male, 12, 25
    See also specific hormones
Hormone-stimulated cycle,
    108–9, 130, 152–55
    electronic pump for, 155
Hospitals. *See* Level Three
    hospitals
Hotel rates for VIP Program
    patients, 72–73
*How to Get Control of Your
    Time and Your Life*
    (Lakein), 8
How to Get Pregnant (Silber),
    45, 71
Human chorionic gonadotropin
    (HCG), 25–27, 90, 99,
    100, 101, 102–3, 122,
    133
Human menopausal
    gonadotropin (HMG),
    62–63
Hysterectomy, 41
Hysterosalpingogram, 35–37

I

Infertility
    causes of, 2
    "ladder of compromise," 4,
        28, 46
    psychological effects of, 3–4,
        19–23, 34–35
Infertility rate, U.S., 2–3
Insurance coverage
    artificial insemination, 150
    in vitro children's evaluation,
        147
    in vitro fertilization, 67, 150,
        156
    pregnancy, 134
    variocele surgery, 26
International Conference on In
    Vitro Fertilization,
    Third, (Helsinki), 150
International Congress of
    Laparoscopy, 54
In vitro children, evaluation of,
    147, 150
In vitro fertilization, 1–2, 45,
    51
    controversies re, 48, 55, 60

cost of, 67, 86, 104, 150, 156
culture medium for, 55
embryo transfer, 57–58, 70, 110, 117–18, 119–20
insurance coverage for, 67, 150, 156
laparoscopy for, 106–9
multiple births, chance of, 110, 151
number of attempts, 129–30, 152
patient attitude, effect of, 124–25
pregnancy rate, 2, 68, 90–91, 158
research on, 51–55
semen specimens for, 109–10, 113–15
sperm count, minimum, 78
technique of, 55–58
See also VIP Program
IUD (intrauterine device) contraceptive, 3

J

Jennings, Rufus, 149
Johns Hopkins University School of Medicine, 52, 58, 74
Johnson, Shari, 96, 100–2, 103, 104, 106, 112, 118, 120, 124, 126–27, 128
Jones, Georgeanna Seegar, 52, 55, 58–66, 74, 80, 83, 85, 87, 88–89, 109, 113–14, 121, 147–49, 150, 153–54, 159
Jones, Howard, Jr., 48, 49, 52, 55, 58, 65, 66, 69, 74, 79–80, 86, 87, 91, 111, 112, 117, 122, 133, 147–53, 155–60
Jones Institute for Reproductive Medicine, 151, 152, 154, 155
Basic Science Laboratory, 158
research by, 157–59
See also VIP Program
Judy (VIP Program patient), 124

K

Kelly, John, 138
Kraft, Howard, 143

L

Lakein, Alan, 8
Lamaze technique, 139, 143
Lancet, 80
Lane, Sue, 124
Laparoscope, 54, 107
Laparoscopy, 16, 37, 40–41, 43
costs of, 72

diagnostic, 53, 68, 70, 71, 72, 75, 77
egg collection by, 55, 56–57, 77, 90, 101, 106–7
incisions for, 107, 112
sperm collection by, 52–53, 55
Laparotomy, 53–54, 78, 80–81
Level Three hospitals, 128–29, 131
LH. *See* Luteinizing hormone
Ling family, 38–39, 46, 47
Lipkin, William, 37, 38, 39–41, 42–45, 50, 69
Long Island Jewish Hospital, 34
Luteinizing hormone (LH), 12, 25, 56, 62, 85–86, 90, 111
Lynch, Linda, 1, 49–50, 71, 72, 73, 74, 102, 104, 148–49, 156

Mazzarella, Paul, 131–39, 140–44
Menstrual cycle, 14, 56, 83
Cycle Day 3, 84–85, 86, 91
Cycle Day 4, 86–87
Cycle Day 5, 95–96
Cycle Day 6, 87–88, 96–97
Cycle Day 8, 100
Cycle Day 9, 95, 98, 103
Cycle Day 11, 90, 95
Menstruation, 13, 32
Metrodin, 154
Miscarriage, risk of, 134
Monash University (Melbourne, Australia), 58, 150
Muasher, Suheil, 154
Multiple births, chance of with in vitro fertilization, 110, 151
Multiple pregnancies
bed rest for, 137
diagnosis of, 136

M

Mantzauinos, Themis (Dr. T.), 92, 97
Maria (VIP Program patient), 100, 121, 124
Marianne (VIP Program patient), 124
Matinecock Friends Meeting, 139
Matter of Life, A (Edwards and Steptoe), 51, 52, 53, 54

N

National Institute for Medical Research (Mill Hill, England), 51
Nelson, Andrea, 92, 94–95, 97, 99, 100, 102, 116, 123, 124, 128, 134–35
Nelson, Bob, 92, 97, 99, 103, 116
New York *Times*, 48, 49, 69
Nilsson, Lennart, 123

Noble, Elizabeth, 137
Norfolk General Hospital, 74, 79, 102–3, 106
North Shore University Hospital (Great Neck), 40, 131–32, 141
Nurses of VIP Program, role of, 98

O

Oligospermic patients, 65
Omni Hotel, 72–73, 84, 148
Oocytes. *See* Eggs
Ovaries
    adhesions of, 43, 76, 78
    cysts on, 89
    follicles of, 11, 57, 89, 90, 104, 107
    scar tissue on, 2, 3, 75–76
Ovulation, 12, 13, 56, 83
    problems with, 2, 38
    signs of, 32, 87
    stimulated, 72, 84–85
    See also Hormone-stimulated cycle

P

Palmer, Raoul, 53–54
Pellucida, 110

Pelvic examinations, 15, 39, 87, 89, 100
Pelvic inflammatory disease, 3
Pergonal, 63, 70, 85, 86, 87, 90, 92, 95, 97, 100, 101, 108, 154
Perry, Debbie, 119
Pincus, Gregory, 51
Pituitary gland, 11, 12, 25, 85, 155
Pregnancy
    basal temperature and, 32
    bleeding during, 135
    blood tests for, 122–23, 126
    chance of, in normal couples, 11
    cost of prenatal care and delivery, 134
    diet for, 134, 137–38
    instructions for, 128–29
    signs of, 126–27
    ultrasound in, 135–37, 140
    weight gain during, 134, 138, 140
    See also Ectopic pregnancy; Multiple pregnancies
Presberg, Harry, 149
Progesterone, 11, 13, 111, 122, 126, 129, 133
Pronuclei, 110
Prostate gland, 12
Psychological effects of infertility, 3–4, 19–23, 34–35

R

Rebecca (VIP Program
    patient), 101–2
Reproduction, inefficiency of,
    158
Rice, Philip, 35–37, 69
Right to Life groups, 48, 60
Rosenwaks, Zev, 87
Royal Society of Medicine,
    Endocrinological and
    Gynecological Sections,
    55

S

Samuelson, Ernest, 15–17, 20,
    23, 37, 69
Schachter, Rachel, 28–35, 37,
    50, 64, 67, 69, 130–31,
    133
Scrotum, 19
    varicocele of, 2, 19, 23–24
*Secret Life of the Unborn
    Child, The* (Verny and
    Kelly), 138
Semen analysis, 16, 17–18, 23,
    24–25, 27, 79, 93
    cost of, 72

Semen specimens, 86
    for in vitro fertilization, 57,
        70, 109–10
Seminal vesicles, 12
Serono Laboratories, 63, 154
Sexual intercourse
    abstention from, 29, 72
    during pregnancy, 129
Sherwood, Genevieve, 38–39,
    40
Silber, Sherman J., 45, 71
Smoking, effect on embryonic
    development, 83, 129
Sperm
    allergic reaction to, 2, 38,
        155
    defective, 2
    hyperactivity rates of, 157
    incubation and capacitation,
        55, 56, 157
    production of, 12–13
Sperm analysis. *See* Semen
    analysis
Sperm count, 78
    low, 18, 19, 94, 151
Sperm donors, 29–30, 33–34
Spinnbarkheit, 32
Steptoe, Patrick, 45, 50–51,
    52–56, 58, 60, 61, 63,
    69, 80, 150, 152
Surgeon, role in in vitro
    fertilization, 107, 109
Surrogate mothering, 159
*Symposium on Male Infertility
    for the Urologic Clinics
    of North America,* 24

T

Testicles, temperature of, 12,
18–19
Tetracycline, 109
Tilton, Heather, 145
birth of, 143–44
evaluation of, 147–50
Tilton, Nancy (Nan)
brother of, 126–27
childhood, 6
college study, 7
goals of, 8–9, 10, 47
infertility, psychological
effects of, 3–4, 20–23
mother of, 37, 101, 123,
130, 141
parents' divorce, 6–7
teaching career, 4, 9, 46, 135
See also In vitro fertilization;
VIP Program
Tilton, Todd
childhood, 5
father of, 21–22, 72, 141
goals of, 9–10, 45–46
Marine Corps career, 5, 7
mother of, 36–37, 72, 141
See also In vitro fertilization;
VIP Program
Tilton, Todd, Jr., 145
birth of, 143–44
evaluation of, 147–50
Tubal insufflation test, 35
Twins. *See* Multiple births;
Multiple pregnancies

U

Ultrasound examinations, 75–
76, 87–89, 97, 102, 129,
133, 135–37, 140, 154
University of California at Los
Angeles (UCLA), 159
University of Melbourne
(Australia), 151
University of North Carolina at
Chapel Hill, 52
Urinary tract infections, 2
Uterus
embryo implantation,
susceptibility to, 157
scar tissue on, 3
tipped, 38
uterine lining, 13

V

Vagina, cellular changes in, 87
Valsalva maneuver, 23–24
Van de Water, Virginia, 149
Varicocele, 2, 19, 23–24
surgery for, 24–26
Vas deferens, 12
obstruction of, 2
Veeck, Lucinda, 64, 108, 117–
18, 119–20
Venereal infections, 3
Verny, Thomas, 138

VIP (Vital Initiation of
      Pregnancy) Program, 1,
      2, 48, 59–61
   application to, 50, 67–69,
      155–56
   individualization and
      personalization, 153–54,
      156
   male factor group, 151, 157
   nurses, role of, 98
   patient cancellation, reasons
      for, 89–90, 100–1
   patient selection, criteria for,
      64
   pregnancy rate, 80, 90–91,
      128, 151–52
   screening for, 67–68, 71–72,
      75–76, 77–79
   seminars, 153
   Series V, 91, 128
   support of fellow patients,
      73, 77, 93–94, 96, 101
   videotape introduction to, 86

Virginia Health
      Commissioners, 60
Vital Initiation of Pregnancy
      Program. See VIP
      Program

W

Watson, James, 55
Whitfield, Margaret, 106, 120
Wirth, Frederick, 147, 149–50
Wood, Carl, 58, 62, 80

Y

Yale University Medical School,
      3